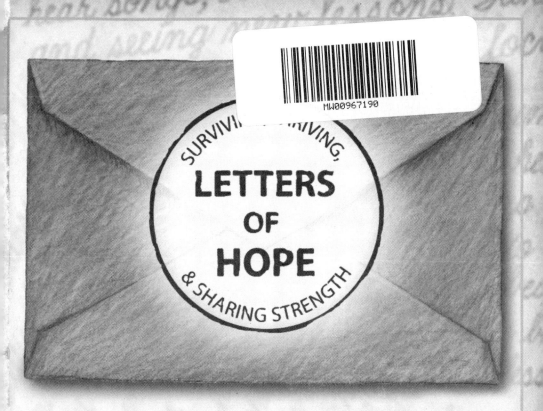

LETTERS OF HOPE

SURVIVING, THRIVING,
& SHARING STRENGTH

by Lynette Carnahan Gray

foreword by Dr. Dan Blazer

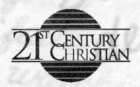

21ST CENTURY CHRISTIAN

2809 Granny White Pike, Nashville, TN 37204

Library of Congress Cataloging-in-Publication Data

Gray, Lynette Carnahan, 1950-
  Letters of hope : surviving, thriving, and sharing strength / Lynette
Carnahan Gray ; foreword by Dan Blazer.
    p. cm.
  ISBN 0-89098-274-0 (pbk)
  1. Gray, Lynette Carnahan, 1950---Health. 2.
Cancer--Patients--Biography. 3. Cancer patients' writings. I. Title.
RC265.6.G73A3 2003
362.196'994'0092--dc22
                              2003019847

Dedication

Dedication

I dedicate this book to everyone who suffers with illness and to all who work to comfort them in love.

Jane

Hope this book brings encouragement to you.

With all my love

Judy

April 2009

Contents
Contents

Acknowledgements

Acknowledgements

Aesop tells the tale of a sacred image that was being moved. With fanfare, it had been strapped to a donkey. As the animal walked along, people bowed to the monument. The donkey thought he deserved the honor. With his head full of this foolish idea, the donkey stopped walking and began to loudly bray. The driver beat him and said, "Go along, you stupid animal. The honor is not for you but for the image you carry." Today, I am that donkey. I should not presume to take the credit for what God enabled me to do. It is God who gets the praise. He took this insecure wimp and gave me encouragements and strength. By using the spiritual nutrition of daily "manna," the recognition of opportunities, and the development of talents, God has shown me His empowerments. I have seen myself blossom.

I would like to acknowledge my grandmother, Deedie Slate Carnahan who exemplified Christian patience through years of various types of sufferings. She showed us perpetual resourcefulness and faith in difficult situations. Through it all, she leaned on her Lord and His Word.

For my Christian education and for the spiritual smorgasbord they provided, I acknowledge my parents, Lewis and Julia Herod Carnahan. For the first twenty-two years of my life they involved me with many types of New Testament Christians: congregations that were newly formed, those in the country, those in the city, mission points, congregations that struggled, those that thrived, and there was even their prison ministry. Mama and Daddy put a diversification of Christians into my treasured memories, thus making me stronger.

I want to express appreciation to my husband and sons for the new ground they lovingly blazed. Morgan never did or said anything to imply that he felt inconvenienced by having a sick wife. Caleb and Boone took each day as it came, without ever complaining. I treasured each prayer I heard the three of them say for me. I appreciate each new skill they volunteered to do and each spiritual lesson they gladly learned. For encouragement on my journey toward getting published, I thank Randy Becton for his confidence in my message and reassurances he gave. I thank all who volunteered to proofread my manuscript and those who enthusiastically gave guidance: Beverly Harwell, Donna Carnahan, Jeanne Ridley, and Renee Gibbs.

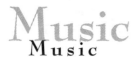
Music

Whether in the valley of despair or on the mountain top, my life and my writings are full of hymns and gospel songs. I choose lyrics that proclaim the majestic power, tender individualized love, or providential care of God. They speak to me of my assurance, dependence, and hope. The songs sharpen my spiritual focus, calm my fears, and change my mood. At the beginning of each chapter, I list songs whose words expound upon, exemplify, or harmonize with the sentiments of that section. Most of these songs can be found in the book, compact disks, or cassette tapes: *Songs of Faith and Praise* by Howard Publishing. Many of them are also in *Praise for the Lord* by Praise Press and *Great Songs of the Church* by Abilene Christian University and Great Songs Press.

Preface

Preface

This is the book for which I longed while I endured cancer and its treatments. It is the heralding of hope through epistles of encouragement and timely information. My experiences with cancer and all that it encompassed reminded me of a high school teacher who read to us from a book that was about the University of Hard Knocks. As sixteen-year-olds, we thought the book was boring. However, because of months spent enduring various medical traumas, adverse reactions, and mental mayhem, I am now a first-hand authority on living through crisis to enhancement. That University of Hard Knocks has bestowed upon me a graduate degree. As I endured, I searched for physical comforts, Godly answers, medical studies, nutritional recommendations, musical uplifting, spiritual focus, advice from other survivors, and the gift of patience. I found no book with such eclectic empowerments so, using information I had written to others, I strove to pen that book myself. I hope you see many different types of helps in my words.

Three months into my ordeal, I learned of two people who were just a few weeks behind me in their fights with cancer. One was a childhood friend I had not seen in decades, and the other used to be a member of our congregation until she moved to another state. Knowing how frightened, inept, and floundering I felt, I wanted to pass along to Barbara and Susan anything I had learned that might make their cancer fights easier. Searching for scriptures, quotes, poems, and songs to uplift Barbara and Susan, and sharing ideas that were fortifying me, I realized that each time I completed a letter to one of them, I felt better. Encouraging them gave me serendipitous hope born out of trying to uplift others (Proverbs 11:25).

News came of many additional people who were fighting cancer. I tried to write several encouraging letters to each person. At heart, I am a mother and teacher, wanting to tell each sufferer some helpful hints for his physical difficulties, some thoughts to soothe her emotional upheavals, and new perspectives to help all those spiritual eyes focus on the hope and peace of Jesus.

Because my experiences were so recent and sometimes even still so raw, as I longed to stroke, soothe, and reassure each hurting body, each fearful heart, and each needy spirit, these letters bubbled out of me. Some of those who received my letters could never write back. A few waited until their ordeals were over and then wrote to me. Others have telephoned or written to me several times. In addition, both men and women have told me in person that my writings spoke to their striations of struggles, giving glimpses of hope and peace. Therefore, my short-term goal was fulfilled. However, the number of reports of people with cancer was escalating. During the two years I wrote these and other letters it became difficult to maintain sending letters to so many people.

From 300 miles away, a letter arrived from Barbara Hoffman Richardson saying she had been reading my letters to her Bible Class. They urged me to write a book. Next, the Ladies' Bible Class at our congregation asked me to teach lessons on what I had learned from my experiences. As I gave that first talk with tissue in hand, I saw the ladies were reaching for their own tissues. Then at all the right places, they laughed aloud and shared my joy. It bonded us in additional ways we had never before experienced. As I ended my talk, from the back of the room came the strong voice of an octogenarian registered nurse who said, "You need to get that published!" Many thanks to every person who has encouraged me to share my thoughts.

My crisis was a crisis. It was painful, negative, exacerbated by temptations, and a quagmire on every level. However, God took it and turned it into good. He morphed it into blessings. Please, read the book in the order that the sections are arranged. I believe that it will be of more benefit to you than skipping around at your first reading. Mark sentences that apply to your needs, and go back to re-read these at another time.

Often I extracted portions of a previously written letter to include in those I later sent to other patients. I explain what worked for me in hope that it will also work for you. If you are currently in a health crisis or have been in one, we share mutual bonds. We have fought a common enemy, but our fight is not only "against flesh and blood" (Ephesians 6:12). Please, read each of my letters as if I had written it to you; I would have if I had known your diagnosis. God knows your struggles and wants to comfort you. Please, let Him use me.

Introduction

Introduction

If ever there was a "Most *Un*likely to Succeed" award for giving people advice on how to cope with sickness and suffering, I certainly could have been nominated for that distinction. Yes, I had sent all types of cards and letters, had taken food and visited. Even though I had experienced surgeries, most of my being had been rather unscathed by truly deep suffering until October 2000. Although my suffering was down in a labyrinth called cancer, it has included negatives found in the struggles of people who have various types of traumas. Like many of life's difficulties, it came in stages. It included assaults to my body, mind, emotions, and spirit. Sometimes I felt that I was wrestling physically against medical tortures and pharmaceutical domination. Other times I felt that it was mostly my insomnia, worry, and inability to concentrate that were the monsters chasing me. On occasion, I searched for a faith that did not seem spiritually muscular enough to support me. Sometimes, simultaneously all of these beasts wrestled with me.

My writings are for sufferers of all types, future sufferers, and for those who want to comfort them. I will tell you some of my struggles for their contrast to my later improvements. Comfort and peace slowly bloomed. My purpose is to give you Godly hope. On occasion, I took out an emotional megaphone and led mental cheers to encourage my own heart. I made lists of blessings and preached sermons to uplift this audience of one—me. I decided that what I needed might be exactly some of the things other sufferers also needed. Passing along useful tips, friendly messages, and funny thoughts became important to me. I will use parts of letters I have written to others fighting cancer. One was a childhood friend; some are members of our congregation; one is my thirty-eight-year-old sister-in-law; and many I have never met. They are your mothers, your brothers, your daughters, fathers, grandmothers, and neighbors.

Foreword
Foreword

Where do people who discover that they have cancer find hope? Lynette Gray, in her *Letters of Hope*, spins a compelling and encouraging story through various genre, including her letters, music, resource recommendations, aphorisms, and recipes. Yes, recipes! Andrew Delbanco recently introduced his book *The Real American Dream: A Meditation on Hope*, as follows: "Human beings need to organize the inchoate sensations amid which we pass our days, 'pain, desire, pleasure, fear,' into a story. When that story leads somewhere, it gives us hope" (p. 1*) Mrs. Gray does just this. All the ups and down, pains and pleasures, expectations and frustrations of her battle with cancer lead somewhere. That somewhere is a place worth going.

Yet reader beware! If you are searching for theology of hope, you must dig deeply, for she does not spell out in neat, logical arguments a rationale for hope in the midst of crisis. If you are searching for a "how to" book on surviving cancer, you will find yourself gratified at times, but you will not find a march step guide to health and happiness. If you are searching for assurance that each successive step in the future will be an easier step, your search will be in vain. Rather, she challenges you, surprises you, tickles you, and at times she even scolds you (Well, not quite, but it feels that way.) Such is her story. Such is the story of cancer survival! You never know what to expect next. Even so, life can be so rich, and your walk with God can be so meaningful when you walk the way of a cancer survivor.

Lynette Gray writes letters. She writes hundreds of letters! Each letter brings its unique surprises. She relates anecdotes, such as an account of her son racing after the mail carrier dressed like one of Santa's elves. (Read further and find out why.) The pace varies and the topics change quickly. Such is the nature of cancer. Such is the nature of hope. "I don't think I will ever be able to briefly mention 'cancer's benefits,'" she writes. "It is such an oxymoron that those two words need much more explanation when used in tandem." Therein lies the beauty of this book.

Let me share with you some of my favorite brief excerpts. On music, she recommends, virtually in the same sentence, "On Jordan's Stormy Banks I Stand" and "Walking in Sunlight." We are not spared the stormy world of reactions to medication, hair falling out, and profound weakness. Yet she finds hope in the future as she stands on those stormy banks of cancer treatment, casting her wistful eye. At the same time, she enjoys the presence of God each day of her life, for she never veers far from His path of sunlight. As books go, she has written a little book, but this book goes a long way toward spreading kindness and hope. On going to chemotherapy, she recommends carrying a strong bag to carry all that you will need. Her bag must be huge as well as strong. Through this book she pulls so much from that "bag" to share with her fellow travelers. On giving a book or tape to a cancer patient, she asks us to consider, "How can a book or tape be the worst or the best gift for a struggler?" How true. How true. The friends of Job gave him a book full (or at least a tape full) of advice during the midst of his struggles. Their gift was about the worst present they could have given. You can pick up this little book at almost any page and immediately enjoy and profit from her homespun wisdom. And homespun wisdom derived from someone who has been there is the very best wisdom for a struggler. A wealth of spiritual insights can be yours as you read this book from beginning to end. Spiritual insights derived from someone who has walked with her Lord through the trials of cancer are among the best insights you can hope to find. Thank you, Lynette Gray, for sharing your *Letters of Hope* with us.

Dan G. Blazer MD, Ph.D.
Duke University School of Medicine

* Delbanco A. *The Real American Dream: A Meditation on Hope.* (Cambridge, Mass.: Harvard University Press, 1999)

Chapter One
Looking for Security

Songs

I Know Who Holds Tomorrow

Be Not Dismayed Whate'er Betide

Master the Tempest is Raging

God Is the Fountain Whence

You Are My Hiding Place

God, Who Stretched the Spangled

I Come to the Garden Alone

I Am a Sheep and the Lord Is My Shepherd

As the Deer

Jesus Lover of My Soul

Gentle Shepherd

My Eyes Are Dry

Only in Thee

You Are My All in All

God Is My Refuge

Dear Lord, Strengthen me to know with all my being that **You can do** far beyond what I can imagine.

John Lennon said, "Life is what happens when you were making other plans." Of the seven well-known predictors of breast cancer, I had not even one. The health history of my immediate family and even my extended family is splendid. Most of them live to a noteworthy old age. As many of my ancestors reached their mid-eighties or nineties, they just seemed to fade away. No relative of mine ever had cancer. Like them, I have always had superb immunity and eaten a healthy diet. With all my precautions and the absence of any cancer predictors that I had heard of, I felt secure. I see more clearly now there is no security in this world; look at the jungle, look at the ocean, or listen to Negro spirituals. Security was ripped out from under me physically, emotionally, mentally, and spiritually as I was told, "You have cancer." Then I was given tests, statistics, mortality predictions, and told to use this avalanche of information to immediately make decisions that would affect the rest of my life, its quality, and its length.

Dear Thanksgiving Day Clan,

In my mind's eye, I see you as you will be Thanksgiving Day—laughing, enjoying one another, catching up on news, seeing how much the children have grown, sharing delicious food, and being thankful. I wish I could be with you. Think of the Russian tale of the poor man who went to his rabbi to complain that he did not have enough room in his little house for his wife, children, and parents. The rabbi told him to also put the cow in the house. The poor man complied and felt no better. He went back to the rabbi, complaining again. The rabbi told him also to move the donkey into the house. The poor man did as he was told. He kept being told to move in more animals. He felt no better about the space. Then the next time he went to the rabbi, the advice was, "Move everyone out except your wife, children, and parents." He did. His house suddenly seemed huge.

We often are not aware of how great our lives have really been. We all have blessings we do not recognize. My friend Martha told me, "Cancer will make you recognize what is truly important." She was right.

Love,

Lynette

How did you begin your day? Many Americans may have begun their days similarly, but according to the American Cancer Society, for approximately 3,655 people, this day will include hearing the statement, "You have cancer."

Dear Roy,

A person can get so busy or so into the usual ruts of life and then WHAM!—one piece of information can change your whole life. Many people will not know what to say during these times, so they just send a card. While that is nice, and that did help me visualize them praying for me, there were days that I longed for more than cards with only signatures. Therefore, looking back on what comforted me, I will be sending you messages of hope and suggestions of things to try to help your body, mind, and soul. Even you yourself will not know what will actually encourage and strengthen you until it happens. So, give all types of ideas a try. Different things will work or not work on different days. Just because a certain something did not work on the day after chemo treatments does not mean it will not work if tried a week later.

Usually psychologists and teachers advise that we learn our talents, strengths, and skills. However, in the middle of struggle is the time to acknowledge and evaluate your fears. Then decide what is needed to overcome them, but do not let yourself live in the land of, "What if...?"

II Timothy 1:7 "For God did not give us a spirit of fear, but of power and of love and of a sound mind." (NKJV)

Yours Truly,

Lynette

Dear Woody,

Disease makes us face many unknowns, but we had unknowns before cancer burst into our lives; we just were not contemplating those unknowns very often.

In Genesis 12-24, we see someone else who faces many unknowns. God tells Abraham to leave Haran and go to a land God will show him. The practical interpretation of this is: you do not know how long it will take. It may be a treacherous journey, the place may be crowded or sparsely populated, and some of your group may die on the way. You can be certain that you will be leaving everything familiar and going to a new environment, new culture, new language, new people, and new obstacles; therefore, take God with you.

If God is going to show Abraham this land, then Abraham will not know when he has arrived until God says, "This is it!" It reminds me of that feeling of being a preschooler in the backseat of the fully packed car on its way to a mysterious place. Do you think Abraham is the very first person to ever ask, "Are we there yet?"

As much as we admire Abraham for immediately leaving Haran and going, someone else has just as much vested in this journey. Not only is Sarah her husband's shadow, going wherever he goes, but at this time, Sarah has not been spoken to by God. Therefore, she shows great faith in both Abraham and God. In I Peter 3:4-6, Sarah is praised for two reasons: for obeying Abraham and for not being terrified over frightening things. This tells me that God understands that not all challenges are created *equal*. He knows what is likely to make us worried and scared. God respects Abraham and Sarah for gradually learning to ignore the physical. Their struggles with relying on God more than relying on the physical are not instant accomplishments. The climb to improve is not even always steady. There are fears, setbacks, improvements, new fears, stumbles, and more improvements. Yet God focuses on their faith that continues to grapple and climb.

Whether we are living 2,000 years B.C. or 2,000 years A.D., those faith struggles begin again each morning. Like the preschooler in the backseat of the fully packed car on its way to a mysterious place, we must try to not let our question of, "Are we there yet?" turn whiny. Along the way, God will supply "manna" to feed you. He will encourage you, soothe, instruct you, and fit your needs. God is able to do more than we ever dreamed possible! He may even accomplish it in ways we have not imagined. As one child in the backseat, I say to other children in the back seat, communicate with the One at the steering wheel.

Hebrews 13:5-6 "I will never desert you, nor will I forsake you, so that we confidently say, 'The Lord is my helper, I will not be afraid.' " (NAS)

In Christian Love,

Lynette

Dear Francis,

Cancer caused me to seek reassuring Bible thoughts. I contemplated a teacher I had long ago who said that the God of the Old Testament was a God of wrath, but the God of the New Testament was a God of reconciliation. Bible examples and my reasoning told me not to believe this since God is not governed by time. To Him "a thousand years are as a day, and a day is as a thousand years" (II Peter 3:8-9). Knowing that fact, how could four thousand years change Him? God controls time. While in the Garden of Eden, the first man and woman did not suffer the ravages of time. For Joshua to win a battle, God made time stand still. Plus, it is God who has decided when the end of time will be. All these show God's power over time. In addition, God told us that He is the same yesterday, today, and forever. This tells me that His nature does not change. Therefore, qualities I see in the Old Testament God are still present in my God of the twenty-first century. Because of this fact, many Old Testament stories reassure me. Even though since Jesus' resurrection and ascension God does communicate differently, I can go to the Old Testament and learn many things about His loving, protective, patient, providential hand working for those who lovely serve Him.

It reassures me that God was willing to play "Let's Make a Deal" with Abraham over the number of righteous souls in Sodom. Even before this count down began in Genesis 18, God knew how few righteous people lived in that city, but because he loved Abraham, He negotiated, renegotiated, and renegotiated again, all to show Abraham how much God lovingly valued Abraham's compassion.

Next, in Genesis 19, we can go to Sodom itself and see Lot, Mrs. Lot, and their daughters all dragging their feet about leaving Sodom. However, because of the great compassion of the Lord, the angels that God had sent took the hands of the Lot family and pulled them out, thus saving them from destruction.

Go to Daniel and see that God closed the lions' mouths. Also in the city of Babylon, we see the story of Shadrach, Meshach, and Abednego who were thrown into a furnace seven times hotter than an ordinary fire. It was so hot that the soldiers who carried the three prisoners in were themselves consumed in the flames. Yet the three bound men of God began freely walking around in the fire accompanied by someone sent from God or God Himself.

Even in your troubles, God is with you. His nature has not changed. Yes, His ways of accomplishing things have definitely changed since the resurrection of Jesus, but God's nature does not change. Curl up with some of your favorite Old Testament characters. Let their lives, their troubles, their faith, their patience, and their eventual deliverance comfort you. Usually, to get the exact details that God wants us to know I read the stories from the Bible itself, but occasionally I'll get out my *Egermeier's Bible Story Book* from 1956. (Santa Claus brought it to me.) These same illustrations fascinated me then as a child who could not even read the words. It continues to reassure me that the God of 2,000 B.C. and the God of the twenty-first century is still the same. God is faithful. It does not mean that you will not suffer. It means that God will discern the answers to all questions about suffering and comfort you.

God is still influenced by our requests, He still sometimes pulls us out of danger, still can close lions' mouths, and He still goes with you in the fire.

Because of Jesus,

Lynette

Dear Willadean,

Recently, I heard a prayer that contained the sentiment, "Lord, keep me in Your will, so I won't get in Your way." During my lowest times, it was difficult for me to pray, "Thy will be done," because I did not know what all that would include. However, I knew that not accepting this would limit God's power and even thwart marvelous things He has in mind for me. My difficulties in praying for God's will to be done, regardless of what that was, were connected to my seeing things from a human perspective. When our spiritual eyes are in focus, it becomes easier to pray, "Thy will be done." If sincere, it is the phrase that opens up vast possibilities. Go to Gethsemane and ask Jesus about the power of that phrase.

May God Bless Your Spiritual Focus,

Lynette

Dear Melba,

Here is an anonymous poem I like. To me its meaning is that if as children of God, you and I pray to Him and stay adaptable to Him, He can turn even bad times into improvements. It doesn't mean there will be no bad time; it means they can work together for the best, such as for our improvement or for a good example. No one's experience will be exactly what yours will be, so let God be tenderly holding your hand. Surround yourself with loving people, hymns, prayers, resting, and Romans chapters 5 and 8.

ANSWERED PRAYER

I asked God for power that I might have authority over others.
I was made humble, that I might respect others.
I asked God for strength, that I might do great things.
I was made weak, that I might do better things.
I asked God for riches, that I might be happy.
I was given little, that I might be wise.
I asked God for greatness, that I might have the praise of men.
I was given meekness, that I might feel the need for God.

I asked God for all things, that I might enjoy life.

I was given life, that I might enjoy all things.

I got nothing I had asked for, but EVERYTHING I had hoped for.

Of all humanity, I am richly blessed.

Melba, I find it amazing that this poem was written by a Confederate soldier 140 years ago. That greatness for which he longed was achieved in an odd way, by his speaking to generations far into the future! May you see your focus changed and great hope flourish.

Sincerely,

Lynette

Though this was not their purpose, these letters became a type of diary for me. I encourage anyone in a current health trauma to keep a prayer journal or diary. There are many different types and styles of chronicles. Your writings will later re-tell you things you thought you would never forget. However, you will forget some of them until reminded by your own journal. You may say, "Well, I want to forget." When you are stronger, healthier, more alert, or wiser, you will be better equipped to use these experiences. Your own writings will help you see patterns, needs, repeats, what frightens you, and what soothes you. Scrutinizing your own words can mature you and any family member or friend with whom you choose to share the annals of your struggles, growth, and enlightenments.

With that same purpose, as I read Randy Becton's book *Everyday Strength*, I used his book's areas of blank space to write my own responses. I jotted down whatever his recommendations brought to my mind: original ideas, songs, stories, scriptures, and suggestions that soothed me in any way. I did not want his book to end. Later, I reread his book, and knew my favorite parts from looking at my notes.

Dear Jim and Kathryn,

Like a robber, cancer comes and pilfers your possessions. We are told that cancer and its treatments steal security. Having suffered losses myself, I want to give you great hope. *Security* is often elusive and sometimes misplaced; we frequently put our security in something as temporary and deceiving as a backdrop of scenery for a stage production. Adversity can teach a person about real security. Besides, in missing something that we thought was our security we might learn that losing sight can develop insight.

Psalm 55:22 "Cast your cares on the Lord and He will sustain you; He will never let the righteous fall." (NIV)

Your Sister in Christ,

Dear Billie,

As you are thanking God for electricity, running water, a refrigerator, and the touch of a soothing hand, don't forget to thank Him for the knowledge you have and your ability to learn more. Thank God that you are able to read and to understand the vocabulary.

Soon after I left the surgical recovery area to be taken to my own room, the surgeon came to speak to my husband and my mother. My dad and my grown son Caleb strolled down the hall to give the doctor some space. While meandering, Caleb and Daddy overheard this conversation.

Two men had come to the hospital to be with their mutual relative. The older man said he had been told that in a few minutes the radiologist would come around to talk with them.

"What's a radiologist for?" the younger man asked. "There's not even a radio in that room."

"Beats me!" said the older man.

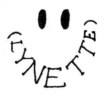

1. Name other struggles besides illness which threaten our feelings of security.

2. In what ways are we sometimes like the foolish builder in Matthew 7:24-27 who built his house on shifting sand?

3. Contrast security in the physical to security in God: how is God more than an insurance policy?

4. Discuss phrases from the hymns listed at the beginning of this chapter which express that God is our real security.

5. Why might it have been a blow to Abraham's feelings of security when God asked him to sacrifice Isaac? (Genesis 22:1-18 and Hebrews 11:17)

6. Name a blessing which you now enjoy that would challenge your feelings of security if it were lost.

7. Why does loss of feeling secure make some people bitter and others better?

8. Explain how the sheep and Shepherd relationship of Psalm 23 teaches true security.

9. How can losing sight give one insight?

10. What in the examples of how God cared for Abraham, Lot, Daniel, Shadrach, Meshach, or Abednego increases your security?

11. Analyze the meaning of the request, "Lord, keep me in Your will, so I won't get in Your way."

12. Make a list of blessings you can thank God for even when you are sick, depressed, or grieving.

Chapter Two
God's Using Wimps and Underdogs

Songs

Bring Christ Your Broken Heart

Where No One Stands Alone

I Am a Poor Wayfaring Stranger

The Lord My Shepherd Is

Just a Closer Walk With Thee

My Shepherd Will Supply My Need

O For a Faith That Will Not Shrink

Who Can Satisfy My Soul Like Jesus?

When My Love For Christ Grows Weak

Teach Me Lord to Wait

Standing on the Promises

You Are My Hiding Place

What a Friend We Have in Jesus

When Upon Life's Billows

He Leadeth Me

Gentle Shepherd, please open my eyes to see how connected I am to Your awesome power and love.

The excellent health of my family meant I had no experience caring for the sick and had not even really seen it done. Besides not knowing medical jargon, I'm squeamish.

Dear Barbara,

I found my breast lump on exactly the same day as you. Surgery went very well, but I feel like a wimp. I'm writing to you so you will not feel alone, or maybe I'll mention something helpful you were not told. During my pre-op at the hospital, I had a very brusque nurse who proclaimed endlessly about my crummy veins. She even blamed her problems finding my veins on me, as if I had purposefully hidden them. So, later, I began asking medical people if there are things a person can do to make finding a vein easier. This is a summary of their answers:

(1) Begin the day before, drinking lots of water.

(2) Be warm all over.

(3) Put the hand or the arm that they will use under a hot water bottle or heating pad.

(4) Exercise right before they look for your vein.

(5) Avoid caffeine.

Each day on my way to the blood lab, I would stop and walk fast for twenty minutes, get back in the car, and drink a hot decaffeinated drink, with my arm under a hot water bottle.

God can strengthen you from: His Word, His Spirit within you, and from other people. May you feel that you are "more than a conqueror through Him who loves you." Romans 8:37

Love,

Lynette

Old Testament characters come to our memories with the end of their lives already in our minds. Kick their final days out of your brain. Go to the beginning verses that tell of the character's struggles. Go with them in day-to-day hardships, uncertainty, questions, and temptation. Now their lives look more like yours and mine.

Dear Susan,

By earthly perspective, it did not seem likely that ninety-year-old Sarah would have a baby. A few months ago I would have said it was about that likely that I would be trying to help someone through the cancer ordeal! I hate needles; I never even had my ears pierced! I remember vividly when I was five years old and adults would ask other five-year-olds what they wanted to be when they grew up. Little girls always answered, "I want to be a nurse." While I was sure two or three of them would make good nurses, this standard answer made me wonder, had all these girls envisioned themselves giving injections! When would they realize the error of their choice? As an extremely healthy kindergartner, I knew nursing requires talents and bravery that neither I nor most of those girls would ever possess. I tell you this, because you are probably not feeling very brave right now. *You feeling brave is not a requirement of this ordeal*—the world thinks it is, but it is not. An observer might think I have been brave on certain days, but I have not; it has been God gradually teaching me how to look for blessings, find comfort in unexpected places, and take every trial one day at a time. I wish I were spunkier. Maybe my writing to you is my type of spunky. My treatments are just a little ahead of yours. Since I am coping and even seeing ways God is improving me, I know you can also cope and be improved. Grab the hope. In Christian Love,

Lynette

Hello Bonnie,

Members of your large loving family who do not go to the doctor's visit with you could hear what he says if you take a tape recorder. Not only would it be good for you to listen to the tape to re-check what the doctor said, but it would also keep you from having to repeat the conversation so many times. Taking a calendar and writing down jargon are good ideas too.

Yours Truly,

Lynette

Dear Chris,

Even though you are a brave and knowledgeable person, your bravery may not look the way you expected. Mine did not resemble a high wire walker nor did it wear a camouflage suit with leaves attached to a helmet. Similarly, your bravery will not look exactly like anyone else's. I believe bravery sees its needs, leans on God, does what has to be done, and lets go of all other burdens. May you discover the bravery God is giving you.

Lynette

Dear Nita,

Beauty is thought to be a shapely body or a pretty face. Yes, cancer and its treatments can take a body part or an organ, but you are far more than body parts. Real beauty comes from within; it is your love, humility, nobility, and spirit. You are beautiful.

Caroline, a friend of mine who is a nurse told me she believes cancer is more difficult on people who ponder. While I believe that's true, people who ponder can be more improved by struggles, because they sought answers. Don't ask questions of blame or what will the future be. Instead, ask: What blessings had I taken for granted? What Biblical examples do I have of suffering? How am I being shown love? What assurances does God give me about His continued care, power, and guidance? How will I become a better comforter myself?

May God bless your pondering,

Dear Linda,

I hope you see God empowering you. This is today's suggestion: quickly jot down everything you do not like about your life. Do not read further in my letter until you complete your list. Your list may be short or long and emphasize the physical, emotional, or spiritual. Did your list include cancer? If you included cancer, this may seem like an absurd idea. However, there are people currently fighting cancer who would not list cancer. They have not faced the fact they have cancer. One cancer patient told me she would not even say the word "cancer." She tries to deny having cancer. Do not deny your diagnosis, but feel free to deny any certain verdict. No one knows the future. Gradually go to the dark places of your mind. Walk around. Evaluate why these fears frighten you. Then decide how you can begin to eliminate those fears, let go of them, or fight them. It's cathartic. Recently, I read this on a church marquee: "Jesus is the Great Physician; have you scheduled an appointment lately?"

During your experiences with cancer, the disease will suggest or scream to you things you should change, initiate, or relinquish. One friend of mine realized that before she begged God for help, she needed to apologize to a friend. Listen to your real needs.

Aesop tells of a merchant who took his donkey to the seashore to get salt. On the way home, while crossing a river, the donkey slipped. Most of the salt became wet and melted. The load lightened. The next time they went to the shore, the donkey fell on purpose. Salt melted. The load lightened. The animal thought this was a great strategy. However, the merchant immediately took the donkey back to the shore and picked up sponges. At the ford, the donkey intentionally fell again. The sponges grew ten times heavier. The strategy which works for one phase of your struggle may not work for another, but don't give up. What was useless for an earlier phase may greatly help you later.

Vary the amount of control you have in your life according to what struggles you are in at the time. Your abilities will grow. The control you seek might be through information, exercise, a support group, soul searching, or spiritual strengthening. Probably at different times each of these should be used. Remember, God cannot use "perfect people." They do not feel the need for Him. Let your weaknesses summon you to seek.

Praying for you daily,

Lynette

Dear Bonnie,

You were wise to have imaging done before surgery. I had scans the day after surgery. Drinking contrast dye on an empty stomach and then being wheeled around the hospital made me motion sick. Step-by-step God taught this wimp how to cope, wait, pray, observe, and grow. Each of those verbs is full of enhancements you soon will be seeing.

Your Friend,

Lynette

Dear Suzette,

You have probably had many different roles such as a daughter, friend, and student. You knew what to expect in these roles. Later you probably became a girlfriend, an employee, then a wife and mother. You probably grew up expecting to fill these roles. However, now you have a new role you did not anticipate— the role of cancer patient. Sometimes fear of all the disease can cause becomes more debilitating than cancer itself. Hanging on my oncologist's wall is calligraphy that says, "God is greater than any problem that I have."

Looking at your new role, you may feel ill-equipped, unprepared, and frightened. I certainly did. Because of drug complications, there were even moments I felt I was drowning. Waves kept knocking me and lapping at my breath. Mentally, I was gasping, paddling, thrashing, and floundering. Through these dark nights, I kept telling myself that I needed to get back to being myself. These feelings made me see my own thoughts at that time as even possibly unreliable. I feared that in this panic, my mind would delude me. That is when I began asking others to pray for God to soothe me. Also, I would listen to hymns. Limit caffeine and don't allow days and nights to get mixed up. You do not want to be roaming the house at 3:00AM. Soon you will ascertain how to calm yourself. Sleep helps.

Do not condemn yourself for floundering. Look at the apostle Peter. He panicked while walking on the water to Jesus, often blurted out wrong answers, and three times denied knowing Jesus. If he had focused on his fears and fumbles, he might have ended his life like Judas Iscariot did. If Jesus had focused on Peter's fears and fumbles, Peter would never have been the one to lead the preaching of the first gospel sermon in Acts 2. Fear tells our hearts that all is useless. Peter did not let his stumbles become an entanglement of doom. Peter's faith can be seen in his striving to overcome and in his learning how to lean on God's strength, not his own. Look for your own very specific victories, even when they are small.

Cancer can change some aspects of your life. However, one thing that you can determine that cancer will never take away is your relationship with God. In fact, cancer can even cause you to improve that spiritual relationship.

John 16:33 "Jesus said, 'I have told you these things, so that in me you may have peace. In the world you will have trouble, but take heart! I have overcome the world.'" (NIV) Sincerely,

Lynette

Dear Diane,

It is a good idea to always have someone go to the surgeon or oncologist with you. This person can help you ask questions. Also, when your mind is going in so many different directions, it is easy to second-guess yourself about whether you really heard the doctor say what you think you heard him say.

During chemo treatments, I had to learn to not silently suffer unnecessarily but to speak up for myself and ask for what I wanted. Because I went to a satellite chemo clinic, the machine that analyzed blood samples was not at that location. I had to stop at a blood lab. I learned that Jeff was the only technician at the lab who was consistently good at drawing blood. Therefore, when we drove up to the lab, if we did not see Jeff's truck in the parking lot, I'd get back in the car and go on to the doctor's office. I would have Beth, one of the oncologist's nurses who was good at hitting a vein, draw the blood, and then my husband would drive the vial back to the lab. After I learned that I could speak up for myself and say who I wanted to tend to me, I had much less anxiety about getting stuck. "Go with God,"

Lynette

Dear Leah,

Your friend Betty Watson told me about your cancer. Betty's son and my son became friends while interning in New York City. Now Betty and I are friends also. You and I have been through similar bad times with cancer. I want to give you hope.

When I was in the first and second grades, arithmetic consisted of things such as 2+3=5 or 7-4=3. Then in third grade math grew more complicated. However, come fourth grade with the introduction of long division, I hated arithmetic. For months, daily in class and nightly in laborious homework, I agonized over it. With long division we were called upon to do every math procedure we knew in each problem. Plus, the order of the procedures and the placement of numbers were of paramount importance to getting the correct answer. First you would divide, then multiply, next subtract, then divide, multiply, subtract, and bring up your remainder. It took a long time. If I miscalculated on just one of those steps, the final answer would be as wrong as if I had done the whole problem incorrectly. In my mind, each step was another chance for all my work to be in vain.

As a nine-year-old with an arithmetic book full of hundreds of long division problems, I was overwhelmed. However, long division taught me to rely on what I already knew, to work one problem at a time, to break it down into steps, to go in the necessary order, to stay focused, that the eraser is my friend, to look for repeated mistakes, and how to apply arithmetic to real life.

One can endure cancer struggles the way I endured long division. Rely on what you already know, work with one struggle at a time, and break it down into steps. Prioritize and arrange working on your struggles in an order that facilitates the solving, and stay focused. The "eraser" is confession, repentance, prayer, and forgiving yourself. The Good Shepherd is having you lie down and is giving you time to ruminate, to look at your accomplishments, your fears, and time to apply to the rest of your life what you've learned in these struggles.

I still do not like long division, but I am glad for all I learned in the doing of it. I cannot imagine how inept I would be if I could not do long division. In like manner, God does not ask you to like adversity sent by Satan, but He wants you to appreciate what can be learned from going through it.

James 1:2-4 "Consider it pure joy, my brothers, whenever you face trials of many kinds, because you know that the testing of your faith develops perseverance. Perseverance must finish its work so that you may be mature and complete, not lacking anything." (NIV)

Praying for you daily,

Lynette

Dear Emma Lou,

There is a Japanese proverb that says, "Fall down seven times, get up eight." There may be days in which you think of your progress and you feel that you have "fallen."

I remember watching my children at ten months of age stand holding the edge of the couch as they voluntarily did deep knee bends. They were preparing their legs to become strong enough to walk. Preparation began prior to the steps, and it took time. As each took his first attempts across open space, he would make three or four steps and fall. Immediately, we would cheer and clap, focusing on his accomplishment, not on his fall.

Similarly, as you struggle, you may trip on fear, wobble with worry, or hit the ground because of impatience. Concentrate on your steps, not your stumbles. Get up and try again.

Like the baby becoming a toddler, who knew instinctively to repeatedly do deep knee bends to make his legs strong for walking, prepare for your new walk by practicing faith building exercises. Let God show you your new potential. Listen for claps and cheers.

Your Sister in Christ,

Lynette

Dear Cayce,

When I give suggestions, I hope you are not thinking I am a "know it all." I see myself in your struggles. In gradual increments God handed me numerous improvements. You said right now you worry all the time. I went through the same malady. Of course, it is much easier to feel well mentally and spiritually when you are not struggling physically, but God slowly enabled my mind and spirit to begin improving before my body did.

Cayce, from my experiences, I would guess that you are worrying so much because you are feeling scattered. You may be looking at the entirety of your worries and feeling guilty, even worried about being a worrier. The next time you get that feeling, do not keep thinking of the accumulation and the guilt. It is like saying, "Don't think about chocolate chip cookies," and of course, you will immediately think of chocolate chip cookies. Take one of your worries that is a low priority and that is something you can do absolutely nothing about, and hand it over to Jesus. You may even get out a mental hammer and nail that worry to the cross of Jesus.

Absolutely insist that you never worry about that specific worry again. Be firm with yourself but only with that one worry. After you have accomplished this for one worry, you may try it with one more worry. Very gradually, you will diminish your list of worries. Go to Jesus' prayer in Gethsemane in Matthew 26. He sounds anxious to me. After cancer announced itself to me, I had to relearn to focus, distinguish between what I had any control over and what I did not, work individually on whatever I could improve, and learn to release myself from guilt. Because of God's astronomical power coupled with His tender, affectionate, personal sweetness, I have seen myself flourish. I have high hopes for you.

Hebrews 5:7-9 "During the days of Jesus' life on earth, He offered up prayers and petitions with loud cries and tears to the One who could save Him from death, and He was heard because of His reverent submissions. Although He was a Son, He learned obedience from what He suffered and once made perfect, He became the source of eternal salvation for all who obey Him." (NIV)

Because of Jesus,

Lynette

Dear Ginger,

Recently, like you, I have had cancer. Even though we do not know one another, I wanted to bring you some hope and encouragement. Imagination can be a curse or a blessing to you right now, depending on how you use it. At first, my imagination kept roaming off to places that I did not want to go. Sometimes I had to put my imagination on a leash. When my mind had a more positive outlook, I could let my imagination soar with optimistic visions.

Fear is a weed that keeps popping up in my spiritual garden. Feeding my flowers of faith will keep those ugly, invasive weeds from getting a stronghold. Just because I have pulled those weeds two or three times doesn't mean they won't return, but catching the fear weed while it is small keeps it from spreading its seeds.

Romans 15:13 "May the God of HOPE fill you with all joy and peace as you trust in Him, so that you overflow with HOPE by the power of the Holy Spirit." (NIV)

Sincerely,

Lynette

In the Bible class that I teach are two very soft spoken girls named Ashley and Christine. Even though some nights they would be contented to answer no questions, I insist that they too respond. Ashley fears that she will give the wrong answer. Christine knows excellent English but is from another country. My goal is to show each of these quiet students that she can be knowledgeable, courageous, and victorious. I would never try to embarrass them. When Ashley or Christine answer no questions, they do not give their classmates opportunities to be pulling for them or giving them hints, they do not give themselves opportunities to hear their own reinforcement of the correct answer, they do not give me a chance to take whatever answer they gave and expand it or expound upon it to become part of the right answer. Other times Christine has given astoundingly marvelous answers that no one else knew. If I did not require that Ashley and Christine verbally partici-pate, they would rarely hear themselves saying the correct answers, they would not feel as bonded to classmates, and would not stretch themselves to act. I believe these are things God is some-times having us do. When we struggle, it might be God teaching us to listen to Him more intently, enabling us to be braver than we thought we could, encouraging us to be bonded to our brothers and sisters in Christ, and hav-ing us witness ourselves doing what we should.

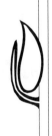

When we struggle, it might be God teach-ing us to listen to Him more intently, enabling us to be braver than we thought we could....

Do you remember that cartoon of the dog who was picked on until he became a superhero? He still looked slow, sheepish, dim-witted, but he went around saving people. "There's no need to fear; Underdog is here!" Do you remember that proclamation? Look at the Old Testament. There we see many examples of God using underdogs. He does not want His people to take Canaan with a huge army and chariots. In Deuteronomy 20:1-9, God tells Moses the enemy armies will be mightier than the Israelites. Then He instructs every soldier who has other plans or who is fainthearted to go home. This will make Israel's army even smaller. God wants to show that it is by HIS power that a ninety-year-old could give birth to a new nation, a boy could slay a heathen giant, and a teenager could shape world politics as he began advising the world's mightiest kings.

Dear Carol Cate,

As a nurse you have medical knowledge I did not. Even though you have been a brave person, when cancer comes knocking at your own door, information does not look the same as it did when you stood above the examining table. Seize the hope.

Evaluate your specific fears, and have them teach what you need to ask God for, to ask others to help you with, to do for yourself, to let go of, to read about, to avoid, and to plan to do for others in the future.

Psalm 55:22 "Cast your cares on the Lord and He will sustain you; He will never let the righteous fall." (NIV)

Yours Truly,

Lynette

Hi Nancy,

I hope you look forward to the mail coming and smile. God's power is best shown by empowering the most unlikely person. If you feel like an unlikely candidate for the suffering and coping, count yourself in there with Job, Joseph, and Hannah. In this time of waiting on God, re-evaluate, re-prioritize, praise God more, establish deeper friendships with people you rely on, and make plans for your own spiritual growth.

Proverbs 3:5-6 "Trust in the Lord with all your heart and lean not on your own understanding; in all your ways acknowledge Him, and He will make your paths straight." (NIV)

Your Sister in Christ,

Lynette

Dear Kay,

I Peter 1:3-7: Praise be to the God and Father of our Lord Jesus Christ! In His great mercy He has given us new birth into a living hope through the resurrection of Jesus Christ from the dead and into an inheritance that can never perish, spoil, or fade...In this you greatly rejoice, though now for a little while you suffer grief in all kinds of trials. These have come so that your faith of greater worth than gold, which perishes even though refined by fire—may be proved genuine and may result in praise, glory, and honor when Jesus Christ is revealed. (NIV)

Since cancer showed its face, at times I've felt as if the world were spinning at a certain speed and I was out of sync. Other times it seemed I was in a trance. A few nights when I was overwhelmed, I felt that time was a protracted panic attack. Sometimes I read familiar scriptures from a paraphrased Bible. I do not rely on a paraphrase for the exact meaning of God's Word. However, because it is not familiar to me, I can actually listen to it in a different way than hearing scriptures I have already heard hundreds of times. Then when I read the same verses in a translation, they are richer. A paraphrase can be used like a commentary.

Of what are you most afraid? For some people, their biggest fear is bridges. They will journey far out of their way to avoid driving over water. Others begin motoring across a bridge but panic and freeze. Therefore, managers of some of America's longest spans now have workers who will chauffeur people over the bridge. Annually, Michigan's reluctant driver program assists hundreds of individuals across the five-mile-long Mackinac Bridge. However, people live in terror of more than bridges. The way to get over any fear is to give the steering wheel to an excellent driver.

You must cross many bridges, but you're not alone. Turn your situation over to God, and trust Him with it. I try to give Him the steering wheel, but then I keep asking, "How much farther?"... "Will this involve pain?"..."Are You sure this is Your plan?"..."Are you really watching and guiding for my best interest?"..."Will you take good care of me even though I have been a selfish child?"...I need to just let God be in control and work with Him. I am always trying to grab that steering wheel from God or be a backseat driver, giving Him instructions on how to carry out what I want. That limits God's power and gets me out of the practice of leaning on Him and accepting His ways.

I continue to pray for you.

Lynette

1. Tell of Old Testament examples of God empowering underdogs. (Genesis 37-50; Exodus 3:11; Judges 6-7; I Samuel 17)

2. Is it true that God cannot use "perfect" people? (Luke 15:1-7) Does anyone not need repentance?

3. List questions that are bad to ponder during adversity and good questions to ponder during adversity.

4. How can fear or dread of the ramifications of adversity sometimes actually become worse than the adversity itself?

5. Contrast focusing on fears and fumbles in the life of Judas Iscariot versus the life of Peter.

6. Using Luke 22:31-32 and John 16:32-33 and 17:9-26, discuss how Jesus taught His apostles and prayed for them that they would not lose heart in trials.

7. Jesus followed His encouragements to the apostles with a lengthy prayer on their behalf. What are the applications of John 17:15-21 for our trials? (Try using a translation and a paraphrased.)

8. Discuss James 1:4. Why are we tested, and what is the purpose of perseverance?

9. How does Jesus' prayer make you feel about your own anxiety? (Matthew 26:36-46 and Hebrews 5:7-9)

10. How can Satan trick us or tempt us when we suffer? (Job 1:20-22; 2:9-10)

11. During the taking of Canaan, why did God not want His people to maintain a mighty army with chariots? (Deuteronomy 20:1-4)

12. Discuss I Peter 1:3-9 and the relationship and purposes of suffering, faith, praise, honor, joy, and salvation.

Chapter Three
Making God-Guided Choices

Songs

Be Still and Know

I Must Tell Jesus

Standing on the Promises

Hallelujah, What a Savior

Have Thine Own Way Lord

Take the World But Give Me Jesus

Hold to God's Unchanging Hand

He Could Have Called Ten Thousand Angels

Guide Me O Thou Great Jehovah

Breathe on Me O Breath of God

Ivory Palaces

Jesus, Savior Pilot Me

Teach Me Lord to Wait

I Need Thee Every Hour

Direct my path,
O Lord,
and show me
how to collect Your
daily "manna."

At the beginning of my cancer struggles, some of the best advice that my friend Martha gave me was, "Pray that God will put the right people in your life." Years earlier, Martha had been examined by a doctor who told her she did not need surgery. Then a personal friend who was a physician came to Martha and her husband asking them to please go see another doctor who was a friend of his. When Martha was examined by this second doctor, he said she needed a double mastectomy. A person cannot keep going from doctor to doctor, taking a poll of how many doctors will vote on which side. Martha was praying that God would put the right people, the correct advice, the best care in her life. I believe He did.

Regarding your choice of a certain doctor, consider whether the doctor will answer your questions. Does he stay current? Does he treat cancer as only a localized or as possibly systemic? What is the record of the hospital he uses regarding infection? What are reoccurrence rates for patients of this surgeon and oncologist? 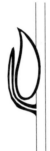 **Pray that God will put the right people in your life.** Does he do this surgery often? Will he emphasize caring along with curing? Does his treatment include hope?

After chemo, blood boosters, and a few weeks of drug therapy had each hurt my bones, I sought a rheumatologist. I waited months for an appointment with Dr. Burns. His exam room was cold, so I kept on my socks and threw a sweater over my hospital gown. Eventually the doctor and nurse came. To evaluate my difficulties he took off my socks, rotated my feet, feeling my ankles, and then he put my socks back on me. I was amazed and baffled. It seemed so humble and actively caring that describing this new doctor to my husband, I told Morgan about the socks. Morgan said, "Well, probably most of his patients cannot reach their socks." Having seen the other patients in the rheumatology office, I knew that Morgan was right, but that did not take away from the fact that my experience told me this doctor cared. He could have ordered a nurse to help patients with socks.

There should be a new profession invented to be a medical guide and ombudsman. This could be especially beneficial for anyone with more than one cancer treatment. It is wonderful that my radiologist, surgeon, and oncologist share files and facilities. At one point during my care, all my physicians conferred with one another in person. If there were a professional medical advocate, he could list the patient's choices, discuss what each alternative means, explain ramifications, or be a liaison among the doctors. Some doctors delay due to indecision or argue over treatments. My radiologist, surgeon, and oncologist are each very qualified in his or her specialty but too busy of course to take my hand and walk me through anything beyond that specialty. I believe an advocate could also assure that preventions are taken so certain types of chemo or the treatments for chemo will not harm the patient's heart or bones. This might be initiated by the spokesman requesting that any patient anticipating certain chemo therapy have a MUGA scan of her heart or by arranging with the oncologist a schedule of a few specific days during chemo when the patient could take CO-Q-10 for protecting her heart. Also, depending on the type cancer a person has, the advocate might ask if the patient can be given the choice of trying melatonin on certain assigned days to perhaps prevent needing the usual bone marrow boosters. (Studies by Dr. G. Maestroni show that over-the-counter melatonin promotes the growth of bone marrow cells.) An ombudsman could also connect the patient with medical experts who specialize in nutrition, physical therapy, lymphedema prevention, psychological counseling, and rheumatology. Your doctors will tell you some of this valuable information, but not all of it. At the present, one of the best ways to learn helpful hints, precautions, or auxiliary professions is to go to a support group where other people can share with you what is available in your city. You will need information from many people to know the care available to you. The role of becoming one's own advocate is much more difficult for some people than for others.

Dear Susan,

We heard that one doctor said you will need chemo and another told you that you will not. I'm sure you are agonizing over that choice. I remember years ago when Nancy Reagan had her mastectomy, some people in the news media or American public were unhappy with her decision, saying she should have had smaller surgery and taken radiation instead of what she did. She gave her reasons, but that wasn't good enough for some listeners. Susan, know this foremost: you must make the decision for you, based on the information that you have and for your personality and lifestyle. People may tell you that their mother or their friend did such and such, implying that you should also. With breast cancer, no two women have exactly the same diagnosis, node involvement, hormone involvement, age, physician expertise, mental outlook, drug sensitivities, and general health. God knows your individual needs. He knows His sheep. Pray that He will put the right people and the best information into your life. That will include your investigations about cancer. Research, decide, and don't look back.

I had a choice between types of surgery. My chemo type and duration would be the same regardless of which I chose, but the smaller surgery would necessitate me also having radiation. Because of my history of sensitivities or strange reactions, and because I did not want to give myself room for regret, I chose the larger surgery. I am not telling you this so you will make a similar choice, but so that you will see the reasoning behind mine.

Right now you feel fragmented, so I stress for you to pray very specifically. It is not for God—He already knows what you need; the specifics for which you beg God, are for you to hear; your articulating them will help you later see God's fingerprints in your life when He answers your very specific requests. A person who asks God for generalities never sees God's answers as anything more than probable coincidence. Also, concentrate on that one choice, your "either/or" choice, not what you wish your choices were, other people's choices or future choices. In such circumstances, I have prayed for God to make His will EXTREMELY clear to me. Gideon made a similar request of God in Judges 6:36-40.

In Him,

Lynette

Dear Billie,

I heard you are grappling with the decision of whether to have reconstruction at the time of mastectomy or not. My advice is to make that decision for you and not for anyone else. Not even your doctor can see this from the same perspective as you. He wants his patients to come back in a year and show how healthy and happy they are. Some women have a husband who will leave them if their breast is gone, or they have such a poor self-image that they cannot get fully back to life without a breast. My husband Morgan told me to make the decision for *me*; he would be my sounding board and help me contemplate the logic of my decisions, but he would not try to influence me. I treasure that! Bottom line: Morgan wanted me to have the best chance of living and the best chances for a quality future regardless of whether I had a breast or not. Much later I looked back on my decisions, my surgery, and my care and have been shown that God helped me make good decisions *even beyond the information that I had at the time*. I think that He was there at that conference Morgan and I had with the surgeon to decide about my future. I am not a person who makes a decision easily or quickly, yet God guided my choice and helped me feel secure in my decision. Since that time I have investigated and talked to many other people in similar circumstances, but I still feel God-guided concerning my choices that day.

As a woman weighs the pros and cons of reconstruction, she should consider: her own age; her lifestyle; medical history and sensitivities; the time she has to devote to the process of reconstructions and recuperations; and how these will affect her future and her monitoring. Research from various perspectives and sources. Get enough information to choose between the specific options you have. Some patients do this alone, some recruit a family member to help, and others learn by asking cancer survivors who understand the choices. Do not upset yourself with an overload of possibilities. At this time, limit your investigation to what your *current* needs are and information that determines your immediate choices. Do not be coerced into someone else's choice. LEARN

ENOUGH TO BE CONTENTED WITH THE CHOICES YOU ARE MAKING. May God bless your choices.

Jeremiah 29:11 " 'For I know the plans I have for you,' declares the Lord, 'plans to prosper you and not to harm you, plans to give you hope and a future.'" (NIV)

Sincerely,

Lynette

In regard to a mastectomy, I heard one man say, "I don't understand how a woman could decide *not* to have reconstruction." "That's right," I thought, "You can't!" No man can truly understand the agony of that decision, and not even women who have considered this only in the abstract can understand. Decisions are so easy when they are hypothetical! Real life has extenuating circumstances, personal ramifications, and unforeseen complications. Never burden a person by second-guessing a decision that was hers alone to make.

I believe God put me in the hands of a uniquely superb surgeon. I will later tell you how I looked back on this and saw God's fingerprints. One thing that my surgeon emphasizes is exercise. This is not only good for getting back movement and agility, but also to help your metabolism, mind, mood, menopause, regularity, stamina, bones, heart, sleep, and recovery. My surgeon encourages exercising while on the bed, while standing, and even while watching television. He insisted that three days after surgery, 80% of my waking time should be spent with my arm above my head. I did a lot of waving, stretching, and just sitting with my elbow up. Each time I went through a doorway, I was to touch the upper facing with my right hand, because that is the surgery side of my body. This is all the more important to women like me, who have had lymph nodes removed.

Dear Donna,

Yesterday as I typed letters to people with cancer, I had no idea that today you would be on that list! A lot can happen in a day. I will be praying for you each time I pray for me.

Prior to your surgery, my suggestion is that you go to a discount store and get some "dusters"—those housecoats that snap up the front. They are easy to get in and out of, have pockets, and are easy to launder. Do not get a size too confining to sleep in. Often they come in four fabric and silhouette styles: (1) down-right ugly, (2) frumpy, (3) matronly, and (4) sweet. Your new motto will become: Comfort and Ease of Movement! (This is where someone should hold up a card that says, "Laugh.") I am trying to anticipate what you will need without taking you farther down the road than you need to be taken.

Love,

Lynette

Dear Roy,

No one person can carry this burden for you; this is a journey each sufferer makes alone, but there are little things that can add up to comfort you and help you see God's fingerprints in your life. Suffering doesn't make one stronger or wiser; if it did, the world would have greatly improved over time. It's what a person does with suffering that draws him closer to God.

One thing that worked well for our family during this cancer ordeal was a spiral notebook. Any information connected to my cancer was put in that notebook. Everyone in our family knew to look for the blue cover on that notebook to find:

phone numbers of doctors, pharmacy, relatives, and helping friends;

everyone who visited; everyone who sent a gift, what it was, and when I sent a thank you;

everyone who brought food, what they brought and when I sent a thank you;

a four line prayer I composed with me daily adding one line and rereading the whole prayer;

questions for the surgeon; questions for the oncologist; their complicated jargon;

names of my anti-nausea drugs and my chemo drugs;

day and time any medicine was taken, and then list any side-effects that came and when;

precious things that friends said; "humorous" things that happened when I looked for joy;

a list of things I plan to do to help other people who are going through similar troubles.

In Christian Love,

Lynette

Dear Linda,

As I recovered from my surgery and waited to begin chemo, I made two non-medical appointments. One was to have my photo taken with my real hair still on my head and the other was to be fitted for a wig. I was advised to try on wigs while I still had hair so that the woman who fit me with wigs could see my regular hair style and color. I scheduled an appointment with her and scheduled my husband to come from his office to the wig store about an hour later. This gave me time to look through the wigs and narrow the field to four. I tried on these four and had Morgan tell me which one was most becoming and natural looking. He was immediately certain of which one looked best.

After my first chemo, I had my hair cut very short. I saved a lock. Then I had my hair washed and styled. When my scalp and even my hair began hurting, I sprayed it with hair spray and left it alone. It stayed in longer than the nurses anticipated. At this point, some people shave their heads. I did not want my head shaved. Slowly, over a period of several weeks, 90% of it fell out. During this time I wore soft cotton knit caps. The hair that fell out would stick to the fabric inside my cap. I would roll up wide mailing tape around my hand, blot the cap, and hairs would stick to the tape. The American Cancer Society has a cap pattern. My cousin voluntarily made me four caps. Getting ready is very quick when you have no hair. As it grows back out, you will get to try several different hairstyles. It will grow back.

Lovingly,

Lynette

Dear Carole,

Your chemo treatments are much different than mine, but what I am telling you is not to emphasize a certain type of cancer, but for the emphasis of investigation. My brother's wife, Donna just finished her chemo. She is the most investigative researcher I have ever known. She scrutinized surgeons and oncologists all over the United States. Even though Donna lives in Tennessee, she had her preliminary diagnostic scans done in Arlington, Texas by a renowned breast cancer specialist whose patients have outstandingly low incidences of reoccurrence. Donna interviewed potential physicians evaluating them by their reputations, their statistics of cancer's reoccurrence in their patients, and their philosophy of treatment. One physician who was recommended to her did not pass her interview, so she moved on to evaluate others. She is a very sweet person. She is not a tough personality; she is only tough in deciding to whom she would hand over her life. Donna was able to find a surgeon in her city who does sentinel node testing to determine lymph node involvement. For her oncologist, she found one near home who was willing to use the regimen of drugs that the doctor in Texas prescribed. I have other acquaintances who have traveled to M.D. Anderson, Johns Hopkins, the Mayo, Duke, or the Sam Walton Center. Each of these chose according to his or her type of cancer. It takes investigation and helps to have a sister, a husband, or friend who will investigate with you. There seems to be endless information on the Internet. I pray for God to put the right people and the correct information in your life.

Sincerely,

Dear Cayce,

You may want to give a support group a try. Some people call them a mutual encouragement society and others call them psycho-social interventions. Many hospitals have cancer support groups subdivided into even more homogeneous sub-groups. Our city and several others have The Wellness Community. Some cities are homes to facilities called Gilda's Place, named for Gilda Radner. Each has support groups for cancer patients and for their families. Their variety of classes differs from one location to another. Examples of class topics might be: Laughter is Good For Recovery, Nutrition for Those Fighting Nausea, Relaxing with Music, Expressing Your Emotions Through Art, Learning to Chronicle Your Struggles, or Lymphedema Prevention. Some branches of the YWCA also help cancer patients through Y-ME or ENCORE. The Y-ME national hotline is: 1-800-221-2141.

While I suffered from hormone therapy withdrawal, I could not handle a support group. I was too schizoid. During those weeks, it was too much information that was mistimed. Even though the comradery made me feel better for a few hours, at night I took all their problems to bed with me. I could not sleep for worrying about each person and her future. Instead, I chose the Wellness Community class in relaxing through deep breathing. Then in the midst of chemo, I stayed at home. Later, with chemo behind me, I sought the Wellness Community again for information from nutritionists and from others who had recently finished their treatments. I cannot recommend each class at every facility. However, I can recommend that eventually some of these informational classes or groups will have something that will truly benefit you. What you find out by sharing information with those in similar circumstances is extremely valuable. In addition, they can help you to know that you are not alone and help you to relearn to laugh. Some people find it truly to be an oasis. Even if you cannot go during chemo, get on their mailing list, find out about their classes and their teachers. Then as you are getting back your strength, attend some of their functions. You will learn all types of information that you have access to nowhere else.

Cancer is the bond that brings each pair of feet to the door of the support group, but admiration, information, investigation, tears and laughter are the bonds that unite the distinct individuals inside. Disease is a detour in your life but not a lobotomy. Just like you, each person in the midst of struggle still has her own talents, skills, education, and background.

Whether you choose a support group or not, don't feel bad about your decision, unless you made the choice blindly. Even if you choose to not go to a support group, if your area has a Wellness Community, Gilda's Place, or Y-ME, give something else on their schedule a try.

Praying for you daily,

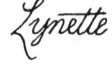

Dear Mary,

Knowing how I agonized over the physical, I longed for spiritual perspective. A year later, our minister David Jackson began a sermon with a quote from Carl Sagan who wrote the book *Cosmos*. In this book which became a Public Broadcasting production, Sagan says, "The cosmos is all that is or ever was, or ever will be." Then David said, "Since the airing of the PBS special, Carl Sagan has died, and changed his mind!"

The cosmos is gigantic, but Sagan's perspective was too small. In order for us to not limit our perspective like Carl Sagan did, we must focus on the spiritual, not living as if this world is all there is. Count on God's promises, see His possibilities, and invest in a future with Him.

A Sister in Christ and a Sister in Struggles,

Lynette

Dear Debbie,

In Luke 16, Jesus tells a very difficult to understand parable. He holds up as an example a dishonest manager who is praised for his shrewdness. However, Jesus says to be like the manager without being dishonest. He has already told the apostles in Matthew 10:16, "Be shrewd as serpents and innocent as doves." In a paraphrased account of Luke 16, Jesus says, "I want you to be smart in the same way—but for what is right—using every adversity to stimulate you to creative survival." Cancer is an adversity. Use it to cause you to come up with creative solutions to make the most of your life. Make plans for how adversity will improve you in wonderful ways you have so far not imagined.

Sincerely,

Lynette

Dear Sarah,

As you are adjusting to new decisions and preparing to enter the hospital, let me encourage you to look for sweet joy and humor even among the thermometers and blood pressure cuffs. While I was in surgery, several members of our church came to the hospital to be with my waiting family. One of those compassionate friends was Peggy who filled the hours with love and funny stories. It had been six months since her beloved husband George had died. They had been a tenderly devoted couple. So, while my operation, lymph node testing, and wake up time tarried on, Peggy entertained my parents whom she met that day for the first time, plus my husband and sons, with humor regarding her life with George. She said he could never throw away anything. Peggy described him as a man who even saved burned-out light bulbs, because he might find a use for them in the future.

She told of a time when they visited a tiny church in Kentucky which was attended by an unbalanced woman. After a series of odd behaviors, when the Communion was passed, the woman took her tiny cup of grape juice and set it on top of Peggy's head.

Peggy told stories of getting toilet paper tucked into her panty hose, not knowing it, and walking around oblivious to her floating tissue train. It was one story after another told by a witty extrovert who is also a voracious reader. Yet often she finds herself with her foot in her mouth or getting into "Lucy and Ethel" type adventures.

Humor helped get this Godly woman through tough times, and she uses it to help others feel a momentary relief from their weight of burdens. God bless your search for a smile.

Love,

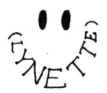

for further thought

for further thought

1. Explain a situation in which praying for God to put the right people and correct information into your life will be paramount.

2. Thinking of Judges 6:36-40, describe ways God has shown you He was helping you make a choice.

3. List additional ways God could possibly demonstrate His guidance to you through: His Word, fellow Christians, prayer, or information.

4. Why are times of struggles when choosing is so crucial sometimes the most difficult times to concentrate?

5. How is not choosing also a choice? (Joshua 24:14-15)

6. Contrast prayers of general statements to specific prayers and tell the benefits. (James 5:13-16)

7. How do you balance between too little information, untimely information, and information overload?

8. Can information overload concerning future possibilities be similar to Jesus' warning in Matthew 6:31-34?

9. Discuss how to handle when you have no choice except the *attitude* and focus you bring to the situation.

10. Use the songs "Ten Thousand Angels," "'Tis Midnight, and on Olive's Brow," or "Ivory Palaces" to explain Jesus' wrestling with choices. (Matthew 16:21-23; 26:36-46)

11. Can a person find humor even in the hospital?

12. How might humor help those who wait?

Chapter Four
Longing For Comfort in the Depths of Despair

Songs

Because He Lives

Come, Ye Desolate

The Great Physician

From Every Stormy Wind

Flee as a Bird

In the Hour of Trial

Whispering Hope

Wonderful Peace

Yes, For Me , for Me He Careth

Precious Lord, Take My Hand

Father, Hear the Prayer We Offer

Prince of Peace! Control My Will

Savior Grant Me Rest and Peace

There is a Place of Quiet Rest

Pass Me Not, O Gentle Savior

Great Jehovah,
please help me
feel Your love
in many specific ways.

I discovered my breast lump myself and immediately quit taking hormone replacements that had been prescribed. In two days, I had the mammogram, ultrasound, and biopsy. Ten days later, I had a modified radical mastectomy and nine lymph nodes removed. My sister Dawn wrote telling me to not look at my scar for what I was missing, but for it being the scar that saved my life.

I was a model patient, complying with all instructions. I healed quickly, ahead of schedule. However, about ten days after my surgery, which was three weeks after I stopped taking the hormone replacements, I began having hormone drug withdrawal. I have a history of strange reactions to pharmaceuticals of all types. This time it was being taken off them "cold turkey" that took me lower than I have ever been. Then other drugs were prescribed to get me through this period, but they brought new and horrible side-effects. Two friends had separately told me that when they each went through this surgery, they felt God's comfort come upon them in a way different from anything they had ever known. I longed for such a euphoric experience. It did not come. I told my sons and husband not to give God any Miss America Pageant phrases like, "I want world peace," but to pray extremely specific requests. Eventually, I got over the drug withdrawal of the hormones, I completely stopped taking the anti-depressants, and my emotional devastation lifted. Part of a letter to my parents tells how low I went. I use it only to show the contrast between the deep despair and comforts I was later given.

Dear Mama and Daddy,

Recently, there have been days I could hardly talk. I was even too far gone to cry. I knew unless a person had seen it happen, she or he would not believe it. When I have tried to explain it, you probably envisioned the me you have always known and the me I was when you left my house six days after surgery. I have not been that person! What I have gone through is the accumulation of drug withdrawal, cancer, amputation, disagreeing doctors, and shaking convulsively from being cold even though I was under four quilts, while my brain and blood seemed to boil. I began to feel that I was losing my mind and that my lack of faith must be the reason God was not giving me emotional, mental, or spiritual comfort. I rocked a lot in a chair that was not a rocker. I could hardly watch television. I had to force myself to eat and to read verses from Romans 8. I tried going to a support group for cancer patients. But then, I worried not only about myself, but also about people who were having cancer for the third time. I was getting one to two hours of sleep per night, and those were full of nightmares.

You know I have a history of strange drug reactions. Pharmacists would have said these reactions would never happen; they are not in books. I am a logical, theological, philosophical, and practical person, but this is far beyond solving in any of those ways. It is the agony of being taken over by panic, negativity, physical trauma, anguish, morbidity, and not knowing how to get out of that place. Meanwhile, doctors went on vacation, did not understand, or contradicted one another. While physicians lived their lives at normal speed, mine was standing still waiting for a diagnosis and prescription. During the short time I took the anti-depressant drugs, you could set your watch by my adverse reactions.

I had already been tormented four days when Dawn arrived for the weekend. I continually begged God for peace. At night I had none. Those were hours when I was dragged to the edge of sanity and received a glimpse over into the land of the mentally ill. As I decided for myself what the hormone withdrawal was doing and what the drugs to "prevent" it were doing, I pulled apart the capsules and took only a tiny fraction of the anti-depressant. Symptoms decreased. I watched Dawn. Her quiet work for us one weekend, cooking, cleaning, ironing, and just being there, turned into God's answer for my comfort on that day. That was the beginning of my learning to look at any of God's blessings or comforts as manna. I collected His blessings, using them for that day, and trying to stay in that day, not asking what He will provide in the future.

I am trying these suggestions: (1) writing down feelings; (2) getting outside into nature; (3) findings things to laugh about; (4) learning how to change my breathing to calm myself. Daily I walk twenty minutes. I list things for which I am thankful. I know you are praying for me, but I hope this explains how specific and intense the prayers need to be. It goes miles deeper than surgery wounds, pharmaceutical predictions, or statistics. I love you.

Lynette

Dear Cayce,

Concerning your comforters: TELL your husband, daughter, or sister exactly what you need. Take joy in their help and feel loved. They cannot anticipate your needs and will feel inept; therefore, when whatever they do makes you feel more soothed, tell them. The first three days after each chemo treatment, I ate five small meals a day cut into tiny bites.

I was so afraid of the chemo, I felt I must be weird. I dreaded needles in veins, dreaded the unknown, and even dreaded the dread. I fretted and felt scattered like a cartoon character who has had his body parts separated and sends his hands out to feel for where his head and legs are. Then someone who had been through this twelve years earlier told me to think of Jesus in Gethsemane; the Perfect One also had fear and dread! That made me feel better about myself. Keep praying that God will show you His daily "manna." In the same principle as manna, the New Testament tells us to pray for daily bread and not to worry about tomorrow. Manna will get you through each day as it comes but not ahead of time.

Yours Truly,

Lynette

Dear Roy,

Before and during chemo, I had trouble staying in any prayer. My mind kept wandering or going to my fears, so I wrote down my prayer. The first day, it was four lines. The next day I fervently read the previous lines and added one. It is no great literature, but it might console you to see some of your own fears in my prayers. Try this with your own needs.

Dear God, engulf me in Your peace, so I'll feel Your comfort and power. Enable me to truly know You are bigger than any problem. Make me feel equipped by You to become more than a conqueror. Help my oncologist tailor all this treatment to me specifically and individually. God, please, take all cancer out of my body. Thank you that surgery went well. Thank you for a loving family. Give me peace that passes understanding and a new bravery. Make my veins, stamina, and stomach strong. Show me how to hand my worries over to You, letting go of them. Put people and techniques in my life that will soothe me. Show me how to grab joy and laughter. Thank you for the Holy Spirit to groan for me, interceding when I do not know what to ask. Please, forgive my selfishness and fear. Thank you that I found out what makes finding a vein easier. Help me to know what to tell people when they ask questions and how to convey what needs to be said. Please, show Your power over chemicals and depression. Enlighten the eyes of my heart and give me wisdom and a spirit of revelation in the knowledge of Christ. Help me see the "big picture" and not get so encumbered with the troubles of the moment that I can't see Your eternal plan for me, knowing that You won't hand me more than I am capable of bearing. Make me feel safe in the arms of Jesus. Help my children recognize good lessons in this frightening ordeal and not get bitter or apathetic, but let us all take this trauma and turn it into something good, giving, and wise. In Jesus' Name, Amen.

Sincerely,

Lynette

Some people so fear blaming God for their troubles that they avoid talking to Him all together. NEWS FLASH: God already knows what is in your heart and mind. It will do no good to try to hide or deny such disappointments. Good can come when the struggler acknowledges his inner conflict and earnestly talks to God about these troubles. After all, doubt can be the doorway to truth if one uses that doubt to initiate prayerful investigation. Neither God nor Jesus reprimand seekers who question. In Psalm 77, Asaph leads the people in a song of discouragement as they wait on the Mighty God of heaven to act. Delays are not abandonment. Go to Matthew 11 where John the Baptizer asks, "Are you the Expected One, or should we look for someone else?" (NAS) John's expectations of what the Messiah would do affected his view of Jesus. Similarly, we also sometimes get disappointed with God, because He does not live up to our warped expectations. Questioning prayers show that you still believe in God's power and love. Complete rejection of God would not pray. The Lord sometimes uses uniquely creative ways to answer questions. These may not include answers you expected, the speediness you wanted, or the method of communication you anticipated. That is because He is God; we are not. Not only is His knowledge unfathomable, but even His deep love for us is immeasurable.

Dear Cayce,

If you have trouble initiating prayer, begin with short petitions uttered often all through your days and nights. Implore God about learning to pray. "Pray without ceasing" (II Thessalonians 5:17). That is active faith that builds more faith. It shows that you want to work with God to accomplish His will. He will enable you.

Lynette

Dear Barbara,

Proverbs 3:5-6 "Trust in the Lord with all your heart and lean not on your own understanding; in all your ways acknowledge Him, and He will make your paths straight."

Everything lately makes me cry. Some people tried to convince me I was just worried about cancer. I could not even think that far into the future. Because of drug complications, I have had trouble just getting through the five minutes I was in.

One night for our family devotional, we read Matthew 9 in which friends of a paralyzed man let him down through the roof. Jesus saw THEIR faith and healed the paralyzed man. So, I wrote an announcement asking the church to please pray for me to feel God's peace and that I would be strong in body, mind, and spirit. I began envisioning, people praying for me. Friends from Knoxville,

Maryville, Hartsville, Nashville, Lawrenceburg, Columbia, and Murfreesboro began sending cards. In my mind I saw couples, classes, and congregations. I saw individuals and families. I saw bowed heads and tear-stained faces. This was how God slowly began to comfort me. He used His people, and He used my imagination. Then my sister Dawn told me this is one of those places no one could go with me; no one's experiences would be exactly what mine were, so take God with me. She was wise.

I wish you comfort,

Lynette

Dear Jim and Martha,

Thank you for your cards and prayers. Because of your experiences with disease, pain, and the unexpected, I feel that you can in some way relate to what I have been going through, even though our experiences are not the same.

I continue to do well with the surgery. As I get over hormone drug withdrawal and the side-effects of medicine to combat it, I am getting more control of my life. Please pray for my veins, stamina, stomach, hyper-sensitivities, and my spirit. Now, listening to hymns uplifts my mind. As I beg God for comfort, I have wanted it to fall suddenly all around me; it has not, but I do see it in snitches, with a little here and a little there. I see it in people, in songs, and in insights. I cherish every word you have said to God for me, even though I do not know what those words were, I have confidence they were loving, faithful, and wise.

Love,

Lynette

Dear Ladies' Bible Class,

My entire family is grateful for every plea you have made to God on my behalf!

My tumor had a rather rare characteristic that will require chemo that is hard on the heart. I ask that you specifically pray for me to get spiritual focus, to have chemo do what it is supposed to, that it will not harm me, and that all cancer will leave my body. Please pray for my veins and my blood cells and that I'll come out a better person than when I went in. I am counting on the Holy Spirit to take your request to God "with groanings too deep for words." I know God is "able to deliver me," but I do not know what He will choose to do. Isn't it great that God's line has no busy signals, no minute limits, and He takes no vacations.

Your Sister,

Dear Mrs. Blake,

Some days my reasoning and senses tell me negative facts and grim statistics, but my Bible fills me with hope. I want to comfort you or strengthen your eyes of faith. God's answers may not be the responses you expected or from the sources you anticipated, but I pray that you will know them as God's.

Job has become more dear to me recently. Repeatedly he asked God many questions. Toward the end of the book, this became reversed, and God asked Job many questions. This challenge showed the preeminent majesty, supreme power, unfathomable intellect, and tender caring of God. Job became so impressed, he no longer needed his questions satisfied; God HIMSELF became Job's satisfaction! Don't give up.

James 5:11 "Behold, we count those blessed who endured. You have heard of the endurance of Job and have seen the outcome of the Lord's dealings, that the Lord is full of compassion and is merciful." (NAS)

Sincerely,

Dear Willadean,

Many people can give you assistance and love, but having fought this fight myself, I send you Godly hope from experience. Each greeting card I received reminded me of prayers going up to God with my name in them. The prettiest cards, I set around the den. Those with the most meaningful printed sentiments I re-read. Above all these were the ones with personal writing. Often I re-read them. Your daughter-in-law, Phyllis, wrote me a personal message and then copied Philippians 4:6-7 from a paraphrased Bible. I knew those verses from a regular translation, but hearing them in modern speech gave them additional timeliness. For weeks, I daily read her card and sometimes several times a day. Phyllis said the verses had helped her through bad days after her heart attack.

"Don't worry about anything; instead pray about every-thing; tell God your needs and don't forget to thank Him for His answers. If you do this you will experience God's peace, which is far more wonderful than the human mind can understand. His peace will keep your thoughts and your hearts quiet and at rest as you trust in Jesus." (The Living Bible)

In His Love,

Lynette

Dear Beverly,

When my son Boone was in elementary school he made a project that won first place at the Blount County Science Fair. He used cardboard, tape, a Sprite bottle, and the tube from inside a roll of paper towels to make an Archimedean Screw as used in irriga-tion. However, before Boone tackled this, he had to understand Archimedes' principle of water displacement. Archimedes had been commissioned by the king to find out if the royal crown was pure gold. Archimedes was baffled. One day as he was still pondering, he took a bath. He noticed that as he sat down in the tub, the water level rose. Since his body took up space, the water had to rise. The story says that Archimedes shouted, "Eureka!" and ran out into the street naked. He used this principle of displacement and weight to discern if the king's crown was a blending of metals.

During my struggles, I often read Philippians 4:6-7. Usually I read it from the New American Standard, the New International Version, or The Living Bible. Each translation or paraphrase shows me some other facet of the inspired ideas. In another paraphrase called *The Message* by Eugene H. Peterson, he explains it this way.

Don't fret and worry. Instead of worrying, pray. Let petitions and praises shape your worries into prayers, letting God know your concerns. Before you know it, a sense of God's wholeness, everything coming together for good, will come and settle you down. It's wonderful what happens when Christ displaces worry at the center of your life.

Did you notice the word *displaces*? It is telling us that Christ as the center of a life will leave no room for worry. Then like Archimedes, we can say, "Eureka!"

Sincerely,

Lynette

Dear Althea,

Do not be surprised if Satan tries to use this time to live up to his reputation as the "Father of Lies." He may find ways to put ideas into your mind that you are unloved or that whatever you suffer now will never get better. Remember that God is more powerful than Satan. God's love and planning for you and your salvation began before creation, and He even used His own Son to be your sacrifice.

II Corinthians 4:16-18 "Though our outer man is decaying, yet our inner man is being renewed day by day. For momentary, light affliction is producing for us an eternal weight of glory far beyond all comparison. . . . Things that are seen are temporal, but the things which are not seen are eternal. (NAS)

Your Sister in Christ,

Lynette

Some people dealing with illness find out all the information they can. Other people do not have the personality or stamina to deal with so much information. While I do not advocate the blind compliance of no knowledge, I recommend finding the level of knowledge that makes you comfortable. Do not let anyone try to manipulate you into seeking less. One lady told me that she once had a doctor who would explain so little, that she stood between the doctor and the door, blocking his way out of the room, until he answered her questions.

Dear Philip and Rebecca,

Use all the information you have access to concerning the type cancer your baby had and thank God for each piece of knowledge. Even though learning scientific information, and taking cancer "by the horns" is VERY good, do not let it become your "chariot." In the days of the judges, God's people were envious of nations with chariots. God told the Israelites He did not want them to rely on a mighty army. As long as they did not have these, it was God who received the glory for their victories. Continue to seek information, as God-given, but do not let it turn into your "chariot." Information is wonderful, but God is our *real* security.

Jeremiah 33:2-3 "This is what the Lord says, He who made the earth, the Lord who formed it and established it, the Lord is His name: 'Call to me and I will answer you and tell you great and unsearchable things you do not know.'" (NIV)

In His Love,

Lynette

Dear Barbara,

The death of a parent during your own chemo must be devastating. You are waiting on God, but not abandoned. Remember when the Israelites were in the wilderness listening to the report of whether they should go into Canaan and take over the land from its giants. Ten guys looked at physical evidence and human logic and advised the people not to go. Two guys looked to

God, remembering how He had taken miraculous care of them at the Red Sea. Their faith caused them to envision possibilities they had never witnessed. Their faith caused them to be adaptable, like trusting children holding the hand of a loving parent, knowing "His ways are above our ways," therefore we cannot figure out His plan. If God were puny enough for us to understand, He would not be awesome enough to worship! No, I have not overcome my faith struggles. I feel like the answer of the person when Jesus asked if he wanted to be healed, and the man replied, " I do believe; help my unbelief." Mark 9:24 (NAS)

Sarah is given as an example of great faith, yet she and Abraham had laughed at God's promise. Then she panicked that she and Abraham were never going to have a baby, so she came up with her own plan, leaving God out of the picture. That was a disaster. Yet we find her mentioned in four books of the Bible and used as an example of great faith. Make yourself use any doubt you might have to communicate more with God, worship Him deeper, and thank Him for good things He is doing in your life that you do not even know about. We were not only created by God, but are sustained by Him on every level. The more we grasp this in our hearts, the deeper we will know and feel that He is God and we are not. Some day He will open our eyes. I guess it will be as if there is a heavenly light bulb suddenly appearing over our heads, with us saying, "Now I understand!"

If you ever feel temporary despair, try listening to gospel songs. They are encouraging to me and may appeal to your musical ear. I just love their harmony, happiness, and the stories they tell.

Love,

Lynette

Dear Emery,

My encouragements are not to minimize your ordeal, but to proclaim concerning the God of heaven and earth. This may be a time when your faith needs a cheerleader to reaffirm the power and love of God. I've used an invisible megaphone to preach to myself. There were qualities of God and faith I knew with my mind, but I had not fully experienced with my heart and soul. Gradually I am being shown how to grow my faith and develop a closer relationship with God. When Paul and Silas were in jail in Philippi for preaching the good news about Jesus, they sang praises to God. I had always been told this showed their great faith. I don't doubt their faith, but perhaps they sang praises to God, because they really NEEDED to hear it, and other prisoners and the jailer NEEDED to hear it. Even though God already knows exactly what is on your heart, He wants you to tell Him, so you will articulate and hear what you believe. Feeding our faith by reading scriptures, praying, and praising God, helps fight our fears. Let your fears show you your needs. After the hymns Paul and Silas sang aloud came a miraculous earthquake. Assuming the prisoners had escaped, the jailer was ready to kill himself. Paul and Silas stopped him, taught him about Jesus, and therefore he was baptized that very night to wash away his sins and to represent the death, burial, and resurrection of Jesus (Acts 16:31-34; Acts 2:37-38).

We do not have to understand all God's plans to be part of them. Even though physically damaged, we can improve spiritually. Pray that God will open the eyes of your heart both as you read your Bible and as you look at your life. The same things I tell you, I tell myself to keep me focused on spiritual things. From my house, your name goes up to God every day.

Yours Truly,

Lynette

Dear Sue,

Knowing your daughter Kendra, I imagine you as a giving person who ponders.

One dark night, when the apostles were miles out to sea on water that was 150 feet deep and in a ragging wind, Jesus came walking across the water. They had feared the storm, but someone who could walk through it was even more frightening. Jesus reassured them. He asked His apostles, "Why are you so afraid?" I very often ask myself that also. Then Peter showed his faith and walked across the water until he took His eyes off Jesus. As Peter sank, Jesus rescued him. The focus of our faith is of supreme importance. Ours must not be a faith-in-faith which is really just a religious label for determination or a perky attitude. Ours must not be a faith that is so calculating and risk-free that it has no "muscle." Real faith stretches, tones, builds substance, and grows. My fears tell me where I need to get closer to God. Some of my fears have to do with my thwarting the Holy Spirit and grace by feeling I have to earn these, even though I know they are gifts, not rewards.

Romans 8:16 "The Spirit Himself testifies with our spirit that we really are God's children." (NIV)

I hope you are feeling God as your All in All.

In Him,

Lynette

Dear Diane,

Like you, I went through bad times physically, mentally, and spiritually, but I did not stay there. Plan for God comforting you through His people and His word. See yourself flourishing.

Not too long after my chemo was over, while I was still wearing a wig or hat to cover my bald head, one day I went to a section of Knoxville where I do not usually shop. I noticed a man walk into the store. First he did a double-take, and then he stared at me. I did not think much about it, just guessing perhaps I looked like someone he knew. When I left the store a few minutes later, he followed me down the sidewalk. He was nicely dressed, we were in a populated area, and it was day time, so I was not really afraid, but I was shocked when he came right up to me and said, "I guess you're wondering why I stared at you in the store."

I tried to smile, but I was leery.

Without waiting for an answer, he said, "Well, you are the most beautiful woman I have seen all day!"

"WHERE has this man been!" I asked myself. A stupid look came over my face, but I thought, "Oh, if you only knew!" My mind chuckled, "Here I am bald and wounded, and he says I'm beautiful! Is this a joke or a pick up? Oh, 'the troubles I've seen!'" There were many things I could have told him, but I said nothing. Under those circumstances, I figured that a smile was enough. Then I ducked into a store that was for ladies only.

Often I ask myself why that stranger said those things. Did I need a compliment, or did God want me to laugh? I still don't know, but I share this to show, life does return to normal, certain moments become more precious, and God still punctuates our days with laughter.

Grab the hope.

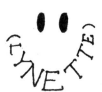

for further thought

1. Analyze how when in the midst of suffering a person may be hit with another adversity that complicates the situation even more. Does Satan sometimes compound our troubles? (Job 1:12-22; 2:3-10)

2. How does God use some of His people to comfort others of His children? (Romans 12:10-16)

3. Compare the principle of the manna to gathering blessings and to praying, "Give us this day our daily bread."

4. Besides the paralyzed man let down through the roof by friends, name another Biblical example of interceding faith that petitioned for the attention of God or Jesus.

5. Explain how the type questions which God asked Job would lead Job to no longer need his questions answered. (Job 38, 39; 42:3)

6. In our bad times, how does Satan live up to his reputation as the "Father of Lies?" (Matthew 4:11; John 8:44)

7. Discuss II Corinthians 4:16-18 and spiritual focus.

8. When evaluating whether to invade the Land of Canaan, what did Joshua and Caleb use to envision possibilities they had never witnessed and to be adaptable to God's will?

9. If God were puny enough for us to understand would He deserve our worship?

10. List things that God does to sustain you.

11. What did singing hymns do for Paul and Silas and for those who heard? (Acts 16:31-34)

12. Why are faith-in-faith and faith in calculations neither as powerful as faith in God?

Chapter Five
His Ways Are Above Our Ways

Songs

Have Thine Own Way, Lord

Come, Thou Almighty King

Holy, Holy, Holy

God Will Make a Way

Glorious Things Of Thee Are Spoken

He Lifted Me (In Loving Kindness)

Savior Lead Me Lest I Stray

Change My Heart, O God

A Mighty Fortress

On Bended Knee

Open My Eyes

Revive Us Again

We Have an Anchor

I Stand in Awe

Holy of Holies, please help me not to give You instructions; keep me in Your will so I won't get in Your way.

3,000 years ago Nebuchanezzar told Shadrach, Meshach, and Abednego he would give them another chance to bow to the idol and not be thrown into the fiery furnace. Yet among thousands of pagans and Jews who bowed to the idol, these three faithful young men said, "Our God whom we serve is able to deliver us, . . . but even if He does not, we will not serve other gods!" Daniel 3:17-18 (NAS) I find that bold and faithful for any age, but especially insightful for their time. As someone dealing with cancer, that must become my outlook. I know that God is able to deliver me from this cancer. Whether He will or not, I do not know, but regardless, I will serve only Him. I need to want a relationship with the Giver even more than I want His gifts. Like a young lady who becomes engaged, does she want the relationship with the fiancé or just the ring and the gifts?

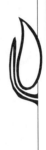

I need to want a relationship with the Giver even more than I want the gifts.

Similarly, in the stock market there is a difference between day traders and investors. Traders make quick decisions to get a fast buck. They do not care about any long-term confidence in the company. In contrast, investors have put their money into a company they have investigated. They are committed to this for years or decades. Investors are not frustrated by the temporary fluctuations of the market. In God's kingdom there are also traders and investors. Traders are God's "fair-weather friends," wanting quick blessings. Those who really invest in God's kingdom are like Shadrach, Meshach, and Abednego; they stay lovingly loyal, knowing that relationship and eternal dividends await faithful investors.

All of this requires great trust in both the power and the love of God. Neither of these qualities alone can give us what we need. Neither power without love nor love without power can rescue us from sin or sickness. After all, they are connected. They were connected at leaving the Garden of Eden. They were connected when Jesus healed the paralyzed man let down through the roof in Matthew 9, and they are still connected today. Suffering is not usually punishment for a certain sin. Sin and sickness are connected because of the fact that there was no suffering until Adam and Eve sinned. Disobedience caused them to be expelled from the Garden of Eden which made them no longer able to eat from the Tree of Life, thus instigating their physical bodies daily getting closer to death by wear and tear, sickness, and injury.

God's love to you has been and is, both initiating and perpetually active. He is still the "Author and Finisher" (or Perfecter) of our faith. Be reassured that a person does not have to fully understand God's power and love in order to use it, be soothed by it, and tell of it.

Joe Beam uses a personal analogy as an example of this fact. When his first daughter was being born, the doctor deserted them for several hours. The baby was deprived of oxygen, causing brain damage. Today, even though she is grown, she reasons like a preschooler, except when she is excited or anxious. If she is frightened, she cannot understand anything she is told. When she was younger, doctors would periodically perform painful tests on her. She had to be awake for the tests. Nurses would hold her hands and feet, but they asked Joe to hold her head. Each time the painful procedure was performed, Joe would see his daughter's longing eyes asking, "Why are you letting them do this to me?" She did not understand that he was letting them do this to save her life. Joe could not explain it to her, because it was too advanced for her to understand. Instead, she had to trust him as her loving father. He could soothe her, but he could not explain it to her.

Dear Carole,

In *The Hiding Place*, Corrie Ten Boom writes about a question she asked her father. As a child, Corrie and her father had traveled to another city to buy watches and spare parts. As they were preparing to leave the train, the child asked, "Father, what is sex sin?" Her father looked at her, but said nothing. He stood up, pulled down his case of new inventory from the rack over their heads, and set the valise on the floor. Then he asked little Corrie to carry it off the train. She stood up and tugged at it, but she told him that it was too heavy. "Yes," he said, "I would be a pitiful father if I asked a child to carry such a weighty load." Then he told her that knowledge is a similar thing. He explained that some knowledge is too heavy for children, but when these same children are older, stronger, and more mature, they can bear it. Then he said, "For the present, you must let me carry such knowledge for you."

Corrie relates how this answer made her feel satisfied and wonderfully at peace. God can handle the answers to all difficult questions, but often we must leave those answers in His care. Even if we were given the answers, we could not handle them. Don't rely on rumors you have heard about God, but go to the source—His Word. Neither suffering, death, scientific discoveries, nor explorations threaten God's power nor lessen His abilities. One weakness humans often seem determined to maintain is living as people frozen in rigid rumors concocted from someone's impression of God, instead of seeking the truth that He has revealed about Himself in the totality of His Word. Pray for understanding.

Isaiah 55:8-9 "'For my thoughts are not your thoughts, neither are your ways my ways,' declares the Lord. 'As the heavens are higher than the earth, so are my ways higher than your ways and my thoughts than your thoughts.'"

God Bless You,

Lynette

Dear Debbie,

Saturday I was soaking my achy body in a warm bath and praying. Then I thought, "I'm talking to God, so He's focusing on me, and I'm naked." I knew that in God's eyes we are always "naked." He is the spiritual x-ray, C.A.T. scan, P.E.T. scan, and M.R.I of the soul.

Do you have a best friend who knows your worst and best moments and loves you anyway? Have you ever been an embarrassment to her and yourself? She might know of times when you got in trouble. She could enumerate your talents, strengths, and unique qualities even better than you can. For all of your positive qualities which she magnifies and your weaknesses which she ignores, you love her. God is even better than that. He knows thoughts of yours and mine that we would be too ashamed to even tell our best friends. Besides this, He knows your many true needs, and He is ready to supply them. God also has a warehouse full of boxes of blessings with your name on each of them.

Matthew 7:7: "Ask, and it will be given to you; seek, and you will find; knock, and it will be opened to you."

A fellow seeker,

Lynette

Dear Carol Cate,

As you move from one phase of treatments to another, you may be pondering causes or wondering how to mentally accept this. I believe it is useless to assume that any person can figure out the cause of a certain trial, whether it was assuredly random, was brought by Satan, or was motivated by God's wanting to refine you or me. I only know that God allowed it to happen. Like Job, my searching to know absolutely the causes of my suffering brings me no confirmation nor comfort. My peace comes in knowing that God is loving enough and powerful enough and willing to take the bad situations and turn them into something good. After Joseph had suffered through years of being hated by his brothers, sold into slavery, lied about, seemingly unprotected by God, imprisoned, and completely forgotten about by those he had helped, Joseph said to his brothers, "You intended to harm me, but God intended it for good to accomplish what is now being done, the saving of many lives" (Genesis 50:19-20, NIV). Similarly, God can take each struggle in your life and mine and turn it into something good. Plan for the good that can be accomplished because of your struggles. Anticipate being more treasured by those who love you. Look forward to having your spiritual focus sharpened. Plan specifically for how you will help others in similar circumstances.

Praying for you,

Lynette

Dear Georgia,

Your struggles have really been stretched out. Often I found that my ordeal was not so much with the event itself but with its duration. The virtue of patience has many facets. They each rely on trust that leans on God. Recently, I heard a new song based on John 11. I believe that the feelings which Mary and Martha went through when they were waiting on Jesus to come were similar to mine while I waited for God's comforts. But remember, if God were puny enough for us to understand, He would not be great enough to worship.

Take yourself back to the first century house of the three siblings. I imagine that at first the sisters doctor Lazarus themselves. When his sickness gets worse, they summon Jesus with all confidence that He will come soon since, after all, He is their best friend, and they have told Him that they need Him quickly. They probably sop Lazarus' forehead and wait, listening for Jesus' footsteps. They probably go outside and wash the bed linens of their sick brother and wait, watching for Jesus' silhouette in the distance. They probably grind herbs or blend concoctions to soothe Lazarus' troubled body and wait for the Great Physician, anticipating His knock at the door. If you could have been there with your tape recorder, what do you think Mary and Martha would have said on the first day of Lazarus' sickness? What do you think they would have said when you interviewed them on the third day? How would their discouragement grow? As their brother dies, so does their hope. They go to his burial. They wonder why Jesus never showed up. Doesn't He love them? Wasn't Lazarus important enough to Him? Maybe after the burial, the sisters wonder whether Jesus realized how much they had needed Him? Was there something lacking in their relationship? Perhaps they wonder why Jesus at least never sent a message or an apostle to explain. By then, I would guess that an interview with Mary and Martha is now full of disappointments with Jesus, God, life, circumstances, their uncertain economic future, and deep sadness from both missing their brother and having misjudged Jesus. Between themselves, the young women probably discuss their disappointment in Jesus.

On day four after Lazarus' death, Jesus shows up. Both Mary and Martha individually tell Jesus the same complaint against Him; "Lord, if you had been here, my brother would not have died." Jesus does not apologize or justify. He asks to be taken to the tomb, and there He weeps. Since Jesus knows the future and that He will raise Lazarus, why does He weep? Perhaps His tears include sadness over what we humans, even His best friends, did not and do not understand about God's ways—sufferings, timing, love, power, trust, and resurrection.

While you wait, when you fight fear, or when you fight disappointment in what you thought God should have done, go to the story of Jesus' three best friends. I urge you to read verses five and six from the New American Standard. "Now Jesus loved Martha, and her sister, and Lazarus. THEREFORE, when He heard that Lazarus was sick, Jesus stayed then two days longer in the place where He was." It seems that Jesus waited because He loved them. We can see that the results were all the more glorious because of Jesus' wait. Because of that planned delay, Mary, Martha, Lazarus, the apostles, the crowd, and all the millions of readers over thousands of years can have their spiritual eyes opened in ways that would have not been possible if Jesus had not waited. When Jesus seems to be "four days late," He is really just on time.

In Christian Love,

Lynette

Dear Willadean,

Over our thirty years together, my husband Morgan and I have repeatedly had a discussion about talents. Morgan is very mechanical and likes technology and gadgets. His profession has been: solving computer troubles, conducting statistical research in agricultural economics, and teaching computer problem-solving courses. However, Morgan says he has no talents. I keep telling him that being mechanical and computer-savvy are talents. He insists that being mechanical is not a talent and that anyone can learn the things he knows about computers. I tell him that I know these are talents, because I have never had them. He says it is all about having an interest. Yes, I know that having the interest is connected to his talent. He cannot understand that it is a talent, because he has always had it, and because he has had to work at it. People are under the false assumption that talents should never take work. Regardless, because of Morgan's talents and interest, he often gets me technology for a gift. He thinks it will make my life easier and more fun. However, I am a person who is technologically challenged. The fewer buttons and gizmos for me to remember, the better. Often when he tells me how to operate technology, I write the instructions on an index card, but then I have to remember where I put the card.

One Christmas a few years ago, Morgan gave me a CD player and a CD. Morgan knew that while I cleaned house, painted artworks, cooked, or sewed, I listened to cassette tapes. Rather than having to keep going to the machine to change the tape or turn over the cassette, he gave me technology that would play hours of CDs without me having to go to the machine. I was perfectly happy with my cassettes, so for months I did not touch the new technology. Finally, I decided to learn how to use it. Not only was the sound improved, my time was better spent not having to keep going to the machine, and the selection of music was astronomically better. I was able to hear all sorts of hymns and gospel songs that were not available on tape. In a way, I had fought it, seeing it only as the gift of technology. Morgan did not see it as giving me technology but as his giving me music. Perhaps when we endure hardships, God is giving us the gift of "music." He knows that it is worth what we have to go through for a little while when compared to magnificent spiritual gifts!

Yours Truly,

Lynette

Dear Sharon,

Between the resurrection and the ascension, Jesus would suddenly appear or disappear. On the road to Emmaus or behind locked doors, He would suddenly materialize or vanish. He was getting His followers prepared to see that He does not have to be visible to be with us! He is with you!

Lynette

Dear Herb,

Joseph Kalinowski suffered from severe stuttering. When anyone asked the boy his name, it would take at least a full thirty seconds for him to answer. Daily he was teased mercilessly. He lived behind a wall of words which he could never speak. Each night Joe prayed that God would trade his stuttering for his arm. Each morning Joe would check to see if his arm was still there, and it was. However, so was his stuttering.

Joseph grew up and earned a PhD. He invented a device to eliminate stuttering. It fits in one ear and acts like a personal public address system. Because of its altering, delaying, and repeating the speaker's own voice, the brain is tricked into thinking it is speaking in unison with another person.

As Joseph Kalinowski transforms each sufferer into a smooth speaker, he sees himself in that person's struggles and his relief. On "Good Morning America" August 1, 2002, Kalinowski stated, "I know now that God did not answer my prayers, because He had something else in mind." May God help you glean from this experience all that He wants your mind and heart to learn.

In Christian Love,

Lynette

Dear Marlyn,

My trials and my readings have caused me to ponder many things. Sometimes, I feel God cares only from a distance. Then I think of the story of Elisha and his servant in II Kings 6. When the enemy surrounded the city with a huge army, horses, and chariots, Elisha's servant was frightened. Elisha asked God to open the servant's eyes. "Then he saw, behold, the mountains were full of horses and chariots of fire all around Elisha." They were not at a distance, but there specifically for Elisha and that situation. I'm praying today that God will open my eyes and your eyes, so that we will see the care, love, protection, and comfort that God has brought in, up close for you and me. I am envisioning myself as a little child held on Jesus' lap with Him rocking me, wiping away my tears, and patting my hands. I feel better, if I help you feel better. I thank God for all the things He is doing that I do not even know about.

Your Sister in Christ,

Lynette

Dear Lillard,

Who would want to eat plain, dry flour and sugar? Who would want to eat raw eggs or drink oil? No one. However, in the right hands, together with time and heat, they can make cake. That is similar to how it is to let God lead our lives. He can take the bad situations and put them together with time and heat and make something wonderful happen. Right now you are in the heat, but God could be making cake! With the weight of our faith resting on Christ and His promises, we will not allow this present life to deceive us or defeat us.

Lillard, I hope today finds you staying in this day, counting your blessings, feeding your faith, and seeing God's fingerprints in your life. As for my prayers, I always pray that cancer will be gone from your body and mine. I have to learn to measure reality not by this present moment, but in view of eternity, and learn to be content in God's hands.

God does not wear a wrist watch, nor does a calendar hang on heaven's wall; God is not governed by time. The Bible gives many examples of God's careful planning, long preparation, the slow growth of His followers, and outstandingly wonderful outcomes! We continue to do fine as long as our eyes stay on Jesus. It sounds so easy, but it is difficult. I think my faith is myopic. I know Jesus can improve it; I want microwave-speed results.

Sincerely,

The apostle Paul assures us that God is arranging and orchestrating events to result in our personal good. However, God, not you nor I, defines that word "good." We often think that this "good" is health or wealth. Romans 8 tells us that this "good" will be our conforming to the image of His Son. As a parent, there were some times when I had to step back and let life's hard knocks happen to my children, because I knew that this would be for their good. God knows you and me better than we know ourselves. He invented you, designed you, created you, provides for you, nourishes you, and gave His Son for your salvation.

Dear Nancy,

Romans 8:28, "God causes all things to work together for good to those who love God, to those who are called according to His purpose." (NAS) I highly recommend reading Romans 8 very often, since it is full of hope.

It was as God's CHOSEN people that the Hebrews endured slavery. Being His chosen people does not keep us from hurt. Instead, it supplies us with what we need to endure. God going with us through a trial can be even better for us than His exempting us from the trial. I think of the occasion when the Hebrews were trudging toward the Red Sea. All their reasoning and senses told them that this great sea would be their death; they would either drown in it or be slaughtered at the edge of it. Go to Exodus 14 and ask those whining, groaning, terrified Hebrews whether they have confident faith that God will use the sea to save them. Their words tell us that they believed they were going to die. Yet God turned this vehicle of death into their path, protection, and their deliverance! Jehovah vertically stacked a sea to show that He can plan the improbable, perform the impossible, rescue the perishing, and soothe the inconsolable. He made the Red Sea the killer of His people's enemies. Perhaps cancer is the Red Sea in your life and mine. Remember the marvelous things God did with the Red Sea!

Love,

Lynette

Dear Edd,

Around the time of my chemo, I told my fifteen-year-old son Boone I wanted him to come up with a poem. I read him some of the quotations that had been especially meaningful to me in recent months. His favorite quote was one used by John Kennedy, but it was written by Jean Hougk, Kennedy's speech writer. It says, "The English word 'crisis' is translated by the Chinese with two little characters; one means 'danger,' and the other 'opportunity.'"

OPPORTUNITY'S PATH

We march on; we trudge with our new leader unlike Ramses,
And in this barren wilderness reigned over by scorching sun,
We carry all our possessions, fleeing the mighty Egyptians,
Their advancing chariots armed with spears, swords, and shields.
They are conquerors of many lands and surely the end of us.
We, their slaves, their property, their beasts of burden,
Are tempting danger, in order to become our dreams.
Suddenly, we smell it, we see it, we hear it, we fear it,
This awesome water blockade that binds us to Egypt.
One million terrors expressed in the chorus of our doomed cry.
We not only see liquid despair, but mental waves crash through us.
If not slaughtered by the sword, we'll succumb to strangulation by
the sea.
Ponder red waters; does it blend blood of dead sons with
mothers' salty tears?

Are we next to intensify this garish, gaudy hue?
Will our freedom flight become its dyeing and our dying?
Our hopes languish—Moses, just a shepherd, led by an unseen
God.
Then the Unseen Breath blows the mighty waters, stacking them.
Grave becomes path, opening not to strangulation, but victory
—becoming our salvation, leading to the Promised Land.
Crisis involves going through danger to get to opportunity!
Go with God.

Boone Gray

Isaiah 40: 31 "Those who hope in the Lord will renew their strength. They will soar on wings like eagles; they will run and not be weary, they will walk and not be faint." (NIV)

In Christ,

Lynette

Dear Nita,

When I returned to attending Sunday morning Bible class, once as I was getting to my chair, I saw an older gentleman lean over and ask his wife if my hair was a wig. Of course it was, but I thought, at least he wasn't sure. Smile. A temporarily altered translation of Matthew 10:30 might now be, "But the very hairs on your *wig* are all numbered." Love,

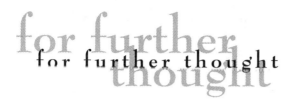

for further thought

1. How were Shadrach, Meshach, and Abednego investors in a relationship with God and not just God's "fair weather friends?" (Daniel 3:13-18)

2. What are the pitfalls for those who believe only in God's love or His power but not both?

3. How are sin and sickness connected? (Genesis 3:13-19; I Corinthians 15:21-22; Romans 3:23-26) How are sin and sickness not connected? (John 9:1-3)

4. Do we have to understand all of God's ways to love Him, lean on Him, and obey Him? Name other things in your life that you depend upon but do not understand.

5. When a person asks, seeks, and knocks as instructed in Matthew 7:7, is the promise for receiving what he wants or what he needs?

6. Analyze the comfort of applying Genesis 50:19-20, "What you intended to harm me, God intended it for good to accomplish what is now being done, the saving of many lives."

7. Tell of your struggles that were similar to the disappointed waiting suffered by Mary and Martha in John 11.

8. Name a Bible example of someone God wanted to richly bless, but in order to receive the blessing, the person had to experience difficult times and learn new lessons.

9. Explain how two people can go through similar adversity and one only copes while the other uses the experiences to mature himself and bless others.

10. Using the example of Elisha and his fearful servant in II Kings 6:15-17, apply this to God's unseen workings on our behalf.

11. What purpose was accomplished by commanding Moses to have the Israelites change directions and come to the Red Sea (Exodus 14), by

having a person born blind (John 9:3), and by Jesus waiting for sick Lazarus to die? (John 11:4)

12. How can God going with us through a trial be better for us than exemption from the trial? (I Peter 1:6-9)

Chapter Six
Letting God Equip You

Songs

All to Jesus I Surrender

Are You Washed in the Blood?

More Holiness Give Me

Father Abraham Had Many Sons

Higher Ground

You Are My Hiding Place

Father and Friend, Thy Light Thy Love

O For a Faith That Will Not Shrink

Faithful Love

More Like Jesus

Stand Up, Stand Up for Jesus

O To Be Like Thee

Turn Your Eyes Upon Jesus

Jesus Calls Us

Trust and Obey

Oh Mighty King, increase my faith in You, so that I will not emphasize, exaggerate, or empower this current trial.

In order for God to equip you or me, we want to be in the right relationship with Him. God is love. It was for each person's sins that Jesus Christ died, but a person needs to be connected to that saving blood of Jesus to receive its blessings. Therefore, the basic question becomes, "Have I been cleansed by Jesus' blood"?

Dear Mrs. Hall,

We have several things in common. Cancer is one of them. I wanted to recommend some items I found helpful: *Everyday Strength: A Cancer Patient's Guide* by Randy Becton and the music: *Walking in Sunlight* by Ray Walker; *Images of God, Volume V* by Jeff Nelson; *Worship His Glory in Acappella Praise* by the Cathedrals; and *We Shall Rise* by Dedication.

The life of your son speaks very well of you as a mother! All mothers want that. My struggles made me long for a closer relationship with God. Even though I have always been a "church goer," done Christian activities, and taught children's Bible classes, this trauma made me long for assurance that I was in right-standing with God. Some people believe merely accepting God is all He wants. Cancer calls us to look at exactly what Jesus asks us to do to grab hold of His saving grace as in Acts 2:37, 38; Acts 22:16; and Romans 6:3-9. Then I used times when I was waiting for physical recovery to ponder deeper relationship with God. Many Americans are vogue on the outside and vague on the inside, not speaking up for God and His purposes and not reaching out in His name. God is still working on me. Grab the hope He sends specifically to you.

Sincerely,

Lynette

In the same manner that Jesus could not be a newly resurrected person before He died, we cannot begin the new life of a Christian before we purposefully repent, confess Jesus as God's Son, and die to sin (Acts 22:12-16). It is immersion that symbolizes the death, burial, and resurrection of

Jesus. (Romans 6:1-4) The sequence is crucial. Baptism washes away our sins and marks our hearts with the blood of Jesus. (Colossians 2:12) This is similar to the first Passover when door frames of Hebrew homes in Egypt were marked with the blood of the lamb. Baptism is the event that marks the believer's heart as belonging to Jesus. Thus when God looks at us, He no longer sees our sins; He sees the blood of Jesus, our continual forgiveness (I Peter 3:22). Baptism is also our way of becoming spiritual descendants of Abraham, thus the Lord's Supper is connected to Passover even for Gentiles, because of baptism (Galatians 3:26-29). Jesus' resurrection is, as Dr. John Mark Hicks says, "a preview of coming attractions, fore-telling of our participation in the future resurrection" (Romans 8:23; I Corinthians 15:23).

One of the concepts that I most often stress to myself and to others is to cultivate the ability to see the unseen and live in the spiritual realms. I believe most of us see ourselves as physical beings who will become spiritual, when the truth is that we are really spiritual beings who happen to be physical for a tiny while. We need to emphasize to one another that we are here on earth as pilgrims, strangers, aliens, and visitors. The song is true that says, "This world is not my home; I'm just a passing through." If your mind-set is purely physical and not seeking the spiritual, God cannot equip you. After all, our real fight is "not

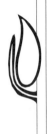

...**the truth is that we are really spiritual beings who happen to be physical for a tiny while.**

against flesh and blood, but against the rulers, against the powers, against the world forces of darkness, against spiritual forces of wickedness in the heavenly places" (Ephesians 6:12, NAS).

In the 1980s when my sister Dawn and her future husband Tim Hammond were students at Freed-Hardeman University, they had a friend named Siegfried who was from Salzburg, Austria. One day Siegfried was very upset over a novel experience he had the night before. He had dreamed in English! This was disturbing because previously he had always dreamed in German, the language of his parents. Siegfried feared that he was losing his ability to speak with his mother who was still back in Austria. Was he assimilating so thoroughly to America that he was giving up his heritage? Was he becoming someone else? He felt compelled by his need to hear a native speak Teutonic idioms, figures of speech, and phrasing. There were no other Austrians on campus and no advanced German classes. So, Siegfried went to the audio-visual learning lab and listened to transcripts of fluid, moving German speeches. Hearing another native speak German re-educated, reconnected, and reassured Siegfried. What is the language of your "dreams," and what do they compel you to do? Reconnect with God.

Dear Wanda,

Just today, I read the autobiography of a cancer survivor who met her challenges with well-written wit. She encourages each cancer patient to tell her own story. As I read, I laughed and cried and cried some more through her story, but I was struck by its spiritual void. The author was bolstered by her own sense of humor, her ability to write, and many attentive relatives and friends. She reached out to investigate, to inform, reached out to take and to give, but it seemed that she never prioritized reaching up. As she went to have her mastectomy, her mother waved good-bye and said, "Good luck."

"How inadequate, how feeble, and how flimsy!" I thought. "A woman is going in for a drastic surgery that will be also the diagnostic guide for deciding her further cancer treatments, and her mother's most effective encouragement is, 'Good Luck!'"

"Oh you poor thing!" I thought. Your own mom is relying on chance and randomness for your outcome. Then I remembered that earlier in the book the author had mentioned that sometimes the only difference between getting to live and die is luck.

Speaking for myself, I cannot be comforted nor encouraged by luck. It is so superstitious, so nonsensical, and so contrary to what I read in the Bible. No, I cannot explain why everything happens the way it does or when it does, but I prefer to believe that some day we will understand and all the pieces will fit into place. With luck this would never be possible. With God it will.

I Corinthians 13:12 "Now we see in a mirror, dimly, but then face to face. Now I know in part, but then I shall know just as I also am known." (NKJV)

Sincerely,

Lynette

Dear Woody,

The things I repeat to you are the same things I had to keep repeating to myself. I kept worrying over my veins, my pains, and the future. When it came to putting priorities in the proper order, I had to pray about it, read scriptures, repeat the logic of it to myself, listen to songs about the proper priority, and be sure that I was not "majoring in minors."

Twenty years ago we had a neighbor named Jim. Being his neighbor was a real adventure! At the time, neither of our families had a spare nickel. We were young and had spent all our money to pay for houses we had just purchased. Jim would often call my husband Morgan explaining what predicament Jim was into that week. The adventure might involve going to a car grave yard, searching for spare parts on wrecks, and trying to make them fit into Jim's car. A couple of times, Jim's requests involved the two of them going to the housing projects and rescuing a child from an abusive man. Another night Jim asked Morgan to help him with a young couple who were having problems in their marriage. At other times, Morgan only advised Jim about cars or plumbing over the phone. However, Morgan had to be careful to mention everything that could possibly go wrong and tell Jim how to avoid these fiascoes before the advice was given. Morgan found this out after telling Jim how to fix something on the water heater, assuming that Jim knew to drain the tank. Jim did not know this crucial fact, and flooded their carpeted family room.

Jim's house had been built by a contractor who saw Jim as so considerate that he would be easy to bamboozle. This contractor turned out to be not only a cheat, but he continued to increase the amounts of money that he said he was spending, and harassing Jim to pay for the work that was not being done. Jim's goal became getting the man out of his family's life. After Jim's family had lived in the house a few months, the stone veneer that was cemented to the exterior of the basement wall began to fall out and down from the cement blocks.

One day Jim called and asked to borrow every car jack we owned. He told Morgan that he was borrowing the jacks of every person he knew. Jim had dug a ditch around the exterior basement wall and saw that while part of the wall was on a foundation, the stone veneer was not. As the ground shifted, the stone broke away, fell down on the soft dirt, and continued to move away from where it was supposed to be. Jim explained to Morgan that he planned to use the car jacks along the complete length of the stone, jack it up, pour a foundation, and re-attach it to the basement wall. Morgan said, "I have got to see this!" Morgan helped Jim operate the many car jacks. Jim built the foundation that should have been there in the first place. Jim's house had a variety of problems, but most of them could wait. Jim and his wife used creativity to hide some of these deficiencies from the dozens of guests they perpetually invited into their home. They never let a thing like that keep them from Christian service, hospitality, or benevolence. They are the most giving people I have ever known.

Jim knew how to prioritize. He did not take care of deficiencies according to what was the easiest to do, the cheapest to pay for, or the most fashionable, but by which was the most important and urgent. Some problems require immediate attention before the calamity gets so bad that it cannot be fixed. If Jim's wall of cement and stone had not been jacked up, mended, and re-attached at the beginning of its troubles, it would have: fallen farther, created a ditch around the foundation, shifted more, cracked apart, become a place for water to collect, and led to moisture and mold in the lower level of his house.

We have had adventures with Jim like no other friend. We treasure them, and they cause us to cherish him even more. Similar to Jim's need, dig down and evaluate your foundation. Today cancer can show you how to re-prioritize with the spiritual in mind. As Corrie Ten Boom writes, "Make God your steering wheel, not your spare tire."

A fellow struggler,

Lynette

Dear Edd,

If you flounder, don't let Satan use depression, guilt, or fear to discourage you or rob you of your connections to God's power and authority. When a person has friends among the elite, the intelligencia, or the royals, we say, "He is connected." Don't forget you too are connected. You have friends in high places. While it is true that Satan has more power than you do, he wants to blind you to the fact that you have connections to the authority and power of the All-Mighty God.

In a football game, the players may be very large and extremely muscular. They each have great power. Without regard to their size or strength, there is a little potbellied man in a black and white striped shirt who knows that he has more authority. None of the brutes can use brawn against this puny guy, because of his authority.

Biblically work on your own link with God's authority. Be reassured that God not only has authority over Satan but also greater power. If you feel discouraged, remember to tell yourself, "I have connections."

Sincerely,

Lynette

Dear Sue,

In that spiral notebook I have suggested you keep, I would advise that you also list scriptures that are especially meaningful to you and quotes that nourish your heart and soul. Re-read encouraging letters. God can be using these people to strengthen you.

There was once a farmer who had a very old mule that fell down a deep unused well. The mule was so old, the farmer decided that rather than spend the great effort and expense to hoist the mule out, he would just throw in dirt and bury the mule alive. The farmer began shoveling. Every scoop of dirt would hit the mule down at the bottom. But, each time, the mule would shake it off, use it, and step up, shake it off, use it, and step up. Eventually, the mule just stepped out of the well! You have traumatically fallen down a deep hole, like the mule did, but use whatever is given you, looking forward to the time when you will just step out of the hole, wiser and improved. With God working on you, your heart, spirit, and mind can be enlarged, and as they are, your abilities will be also.

Your Sister,

Dear Herb,

In the play *As You Like It*, William Shakespeare writes that the uses of adversity can be sweet, enabling one to find "tongues in trees, books in brooks, and sermons in stones." I would guess that as you look around at God's creation, as you read scriptures, hear songs, or listen to conversations, you are hearing and seeing new lessons. Take note of them and cherish your sharpened spiritual vision.

In Christian Love,

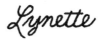

Dear Kay,

Over the years, I have heard thousands of sermons and hundreds of Bible lessons at Christian schools, but now I am getting new lessons from a variety of Bible verses, not because the Bible has changed or now says more; I am seeing new things, because I have changed. I have new eyes and an expanded heart—that of someone touched by suffering. Like Helen Keller said, "When one door of happiness closes, another will open; often we look so long at the closed door that we do not see the one God has opened to us." I believe some of my usual doors of happiness closed when cancer came, but God has opened other doors of a more mature kind of happiness. I hope you are seeing newly opened doors.

In Him,

Lynette

Taking any type of action helps me feel like less of a victim. The action gives me hope. My first action was the prayers I kept saying to God and then asking other Christians to pray for me. After surgery I took the action of doing exercises and walking for twenty minutes a day. I walked fast to the beat of each hymn that I sang: "Walking in Sunlight," "One Step at a Time," "Hold to God's Unchanging Hand," "Leaning on the Everlasting Arms," "Anywhere With Jesus," and "We're Marching to Zion." Next, I took the action of reaching out to others by asking my friend Beverly to be a liaison for me to our congregation. I conducted my own personal survey asking several medical people what could make finding a vein easier. As people sent me gifts, letters, food, and flowers, I took the action to write them thank you notes that included asking for continuing prayers. I kept a list of any prescriptions or I.V. drugs I was given, their timetable, and then any reactions. This proved profitable to substantiate drug-induced problems. I went to the Wellness Community to learn how to relax with deep breathing. I researched cancer and thought up questions to ask the doctor, but only in the mornings. Studying cancer late in the day tended to mean that I would take those thoughts to bed with me. The weather turned cold and the wind grew severe. I mentioned to my friend Beverly that I wished I could exercise indoors. Beverly loaned me a stationary bike. I was delighted. My next action was to ride that stationary bike. I would put on the hymns, pedal and sing, pedal and pray, and sing, and cry. I thanked God that I was able to cry; there had been a time when I was so "far gone," that I did not even cry. I knew that once I was able to cry again, things were getting better. Besides, as I explained to my sons and husband, there are many different types of crying. Some of them are very therapeutic. At a couple of stages during the various problems I have come through, I had difficulty sleeping. During those hours, listening to hymns on my headphones was again the best action I could take. It seems to ground and soothe me.

My warning to patients is, do not measure yourself by your productivity right now. On highway 109, near Gallatin, our friend Jim was hit by a drunk driver and at death's door. After innumerable prayers, several surgeries, and weeks of rest, Jim was visited by a certain friend. Jim told the man that because he could not do anything, he felt useless to his family. Jim's friend told him, "This may be exactly what your family needs to see right now!"

When the Good Shepherd has us lie down, it is time to ruminate: ponder, pray, sing, cry, read, and reach out. Leslie, a quiet young lady in our congregation, sent me a prayer diary. I hardly knew her, but having gone through pain herself is probably what prompted her to send me this gift. It not only has space to write prayers, but it also asks questions. This is a superb time to be asking questions and praying for answers, re-prioritizing and planning how to comfort others.

Dear Ellen,

I hope you do not think this letter is narcissistic, but giving you personal examples helps me explain the new territory you are entering. As a child, teenager, and young adult, I generally never defended myself against intimidating people or situations. I would avoid such or get out of that type situation. I remember being over-charged, over-looked, and misunderstood, but I said nothing to the store clerk, teachers, or other adults who occasionally treated me wrongly. Then came motherhood. Eventually, my precious little ones went to school. When anyone, no matter how big, important, or knowledgeable that person might be, mistreated, over-looked, or misunderstood my child, I was there with a thorough, logical, loving, comprehensive defense, new strategy, and how to implement the plan. Ellen, I imagine you also as a very loving mother who would do anything necessary to protect and comfort her children. The person whom you most need to nurture, soothe, comfort, and strengthen now is you! Become your own child; occasionally remove yourself from being you; ask yourself what Ellen deeply needs. Find times to imagine how it is to look at you from God's perspective. The trauma of all this has made me long for a closer, deeper relationship with God. I am praying for you.

Grab the hope,

Lynette

Dear Cayce,

Your letter concerning emotions tells me that perhaps you are on overload. This may be for two reasons: (1) you have many people depending on you; and (2) you have prioritized some things that should not have top priority. I cannot tell you what those issues are, but I would guess that in certain areas, you have majored in minors. Let go of some of your self-imposed burdens. For example: at the beginning of my chemo, I taught my husband how to clean the bathroom. Also, when my fifteen-year-old son had a conflict with one teacher at his high school, I told my family I could not step in and be his spokesman the way I had always been. Therefore, our older son Caleb said he would deal with the situation. I applauded Caleb as he contacted the chairman of the department and the school principal on behalf of his brother. I sat back very proud of Caleb as he composed an articulate explanation of why his brother's treatment had been both unjust and invalid. The grade was changed. My point is, if I had not given up some of my usual activities, neither my husband nor our older son would have taken on these responsibilities. During my chemo, it was not selfish of me to let others meet these needs. Instead, it allowed them to grow, give, sympathize, and experience things I had been the only one to do. Sometimes in these circumstances, the wisest action that you can do is to help someone else learn how to do it.

God bless your heart and mind,

Lynette

Hello Suzette,

I will tell you one of the unusual things I ordered from the American Cancer Society catalog. For when I wanted to wear a soft hat or scarf instead of my wig, I bought bangs. This was a strip of hair fringe sewn to a stretchy headband. Since I had nothing to hang out from under a hat, the bangs made me look more normal without being too tight or itchy. They are an inexpensive change that might perk up your looks. They sure did a lot for mine.

No one warned me about a certain side effect of chemo, nor did I read of it in any of the literature given to me. However, it did happen to me for a short time. As chemo progressed, I would find myself sometimes having difficulty thinking of a certain word, or I might begin a sentence and forget where I was going with it. My husband says that for a short while, I was more affected than I realized. This malady is called "chemo brain."

One lady to whom I write says that during her days in chemo brain, she would pick up a mail order catalog that had come a day earlier and see certain items that had been marked. She would know that she had been the one who marked those items, but she could not figure out why in the world these articles had ever interested her. She knew that it was the mystery of chemo brain, but she never expected it to manifest itself in ways so uncharacteristic of her.

As for my own personal experience, my brain was actually more affected later by an anti-estrogen than it was by the chemo. I was quickly taken off the drug. Time and very good nutrition took away the drug's effects on my mind. For whenever chemo is totally completed, I stress the most nutritious foods and the proper supplementation which should include trace minerals. Chemo and other treatments greatly deplete more of your health than anyone seems to discuss. Taking action to study optimal nutrition and learning how to get it, will greatly help you not only get rid of chemo brain but even also become possibly healthier than you were in the past!

May God bless your investigations.

Lynette

Dear Susan,

Romans 8:18 "What we suffer now is nothing compared to the glory He will give us later."

I wanted to tell you the reasons I wrote down each medicine I took and symptoms each brought. **(1)** I just scribbled down in my spiral notebook and later typed them, so I would have a copy to give the doctor to ask him if I was reacting as expected or if something should be changed. **(2)** My mind was too foggy to go back later and try to remember when what happened, but if I had written it down, I could trust that validation. **(3)** If something out of the ordinary happened, I could look back at my time-table and figure out the cause. In the case of one anti-nausea drug, it gave me the first migraine headache I had ever had in my life, so the doctor substituted for a different drug. **(4)** The day I was given chemo treatments was called Day 1, and then the days of each cycle were numbered. Subsequent cycles if I had diarrhea or my eyes hurt, I could look back and see that on the previous cycle on that certain day, the same symptom came. Then I would look for when it went away. When I could see symptoms that stopped in one or two days, that gave me hope. **(5)** In some way, keeping the chart puts a little more control back into your life, rather than not being able to see causes and effects and anticipate improvements.

I would not do cancer the honor of naming a computer file after it. Also, I did not want a constant reminder of cancer's negatives. So, all these things are in one of my computer files that I named "cure."

In Christian Love,

Lynette

Dear Linda,

One of my friends who had breast cancer and a mastectomy twenty-one years ago often tells this scene from her life. I will call this lady Eve. When Eve first found out that she had breast cancer, she tells that she asked God why He would let a woman who was not so abundantly endowed in the first place be one who had to have her breast removed. Then while Eve was still in the hospital from having had her mastectomy, a young lady came to visit her, looked at Eve's chest and asked, "Which side was it?" Eve still laughs about that. Some people would think that the focus of that statement is that Eve was small breasted or that well-intentioned people sometimes say the wrong things. In contrast, I believe that the focus should be that because Eve did laugh and still laughs about it, is one of the reasons why she is still "alive and kickin" twenty-one years later. Find any excuse you can to laugh!

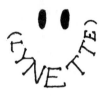

for further thought

for further thought

1. Why is relationship with God important? (Matthew 7:21; Luke 15:17-24; Acts 17:24-31; Philippians 3:13-15)

2. In becoming a Christian, what represents Christ's death, burial, and resurrection? (Romans 6:3-6)

3. Can a person rise to a new life before he has died to sin and been buried in baptism with Christ? Why was and is *sequence* important? (Colossians 2:8-14; Galatians 3:27; I Peter 3:18-21)

4. How does obedient faith make us spiritual descendants of Abraham? (Romans 4:16-18)

5. What is the connection of the Lord's Supper to the Passover?

6. Name songs which speak to the fact that Christians are here as pilgrims, strangers, and aliens.

7. How is a struggle with finances, bereavement, health, depression, or relationships also a fight against the forces of wickedness? (Ephesians 6:12)

8. In what ways do we use God as our spare tire instead of our steering wheel?

9. How does adversity help us find "tongues in trees, books in brooks, and sermons in stones"?

10. In Psalm 23, who insisted that the sheep lie down? Why?

11. What was the most frightening place the sheep went? Why did this not terrify him?

12. How do Hebrews 12:5-11 and the words to the song "O For a Faith That Will Not Shrink" tell us that even though we cannot understand God's ways His purposes are to equip us?

Chapter Seven
Helping a Child Understand Suffering

Songs

No One Ever Cared for Me Like Jesus

Can You Count the Stars of Evening?

Tell Me the Old, Old Story

It Is Well With My Soul

Jesus Loves Me

Jesus Friend of Children

He Is Able

Does Jesus Care?

Jesus Loves Even Me

Just a Little Talk With Jesus

Jesus Loves the Little Children

Immortal, Invisible, God Only Wise

Dear Heavenly Father, please **give me the words** to explain to a child Your blessings of **love, power, and hope** for those who serve You.

Without being negative or melancholy, even children need to know life is sometimes not fair. I remember incidences when my own children lamented over an unfairness in their lives because there was a person who treated them unkindly. The child treated unjustly needed sympathy at that moment, so I would acknowledge, "Yes, this was unfair; you deserved better." However, I would then say, "Just as this was an unfair situation today, and you did not get what you deserved, there have been other times in your past when you received *better* than you deserved. Perhaps a person responded to you graciously after you had been thoughtless, or you might have placed higher in a contest than you deserved. Remember, the fact that life is not always fair has two sides. Sometimes you get worse than you earned, but other times you have received better than you deserved. My friend Kym Lain tells her children, 'No, life is not fair. Fair is another name for an amusement park.'"

God is not ruled by any limited view of political fairness. His view is more than astronomically larger than ours. You are so much more than just a body, therefore His view of you includes His tender love for your eternal soul. Since your soul will last much longer than your body, if using lessons through the body will enable your soul to dwell in heaven, it will be worth the pain.

The Spanish artist Pablo Picasso could not read English. Therefore, he said that for him, written English made no sense, but he went on to say that even though he could not read it, he knew that it still had meaning and reason. He believed in something he could not understand. Similarly, I do not understand how signals or waves of light and sound come through the air and become television programs, yet I still watch television. On a FAR grander scale, even though I do not understand many aspects of God, He is still to be worshiped. I believe that God will eventually show us that He is even better than our idea of fair. We must teach our children to treasure His supreme love that asks us to faithfully wait for the explanation.

The fact that sometimes small children suffer is especially perplexing. It makes no sense now, because we are still looking "through a glass darkly" (I Corinthians 13:12). Our limited knowledge prevents us from understanding. Be reassured that someday we will understand it. The following is a letter I wrote to a seven-year-old with bone cancer.

Dear Brendle,

I am a friend of your gymnastics teammate Emily Jones. Her mom Vicki told us you have cancer. Two years ago, when I found out I had cancer, I had to stop doing many things that I was used to doing, because the medicine made me weak and made me unable to fight off germs. Therefore, I had to stay at the hospital a few days and at home several months. But, even when I had cancer, one of the few things that I did not have to stop doing was—praying. At first, I was upset by all the places I would not be able to go and the things I would not be able to do. If I had concentrated on what I was missing, I would have become mad and sad. Instead, I decided to talk about all the things that I was thankful for even in the bad times. While I felt so weak, I counted all the good things I had noticed and appreciated. In many foreign countries when a person gets sick, she has no wonderful hospitals. So, I thanked God for great hospitals, smart doctors, those who love me, for a car that worked, and even for clean sheets and clean water. Sometimes I wrote down these good things. They are called blessings.

The doctor that decided which medicines I should take and who looked at how healthy my blood was is named Dr. Brig. One thing that helped him be a good doctor is that when he was a kid, he had cancer. Like you, he had been a gymnast! His treatments for cancer made him weak, but today he has no cancer. Plus, because of having cancer, he knows how it feels. He really cares and we call that compassion.

The medicine I took made my hair fall out. I looked pale with no hair, so I liked to wear bright colors. Red, blue, and pink made me look the best, so I am sending you a bandana with those colors and more. You can wear it with nothing else on your head, or wear it with a baseball cap. I thought the shoes pictured on the fabric were just what a girl your age should have.

These days I am no longer weak, I have no cancer, and I have lots of hair. I am praying for you.

Your friend,

Lynette Gray

Dear Beverly,

Perhaps as people of science and technology, something as mysterious as prayer baffles us so much that we do not make enough use of its power and the relationship it brings. Besides the great need I felt for the intercessory prayers of fellow Christians and the deep need to improve my own prayers, I had another lesson to learn about prayer. This lesson came through a child. After months of being away from teaching my girls' Bible class, the girls kept inquiring of their substitute teacher Nina and others asking when I would return. I had counted up the surgery, its recuperation, chemo, and more recuperation and estimated when I would be back. When spring came, and I was not back in class, the girls worried that I would never return. A few months later when I did feel well enough to resume teaching, I knew they wanted an explanation of why I had forsaken them so long. Without giving them details that would frighten them or that were too much information, I explained what I had been through emphasizing God guiding me, enabling me, and improving me. I discussed my prayers and those of other people for me. I told the girls that I cherished even children's prayers—especially children's prayers. When I finished speaking about the fact that sometimes God's answer is, "Wait," an eight-year-old named Erin raised her hand. She told the class and me that the previous year when she had lived in another city, she had a Bible class teacher who told her this experience. For years the lady had prayed about a specific need and saw no results, but she continued asking God. Then His affirming answer came. It had been fifteen years since the woman's pleas began! It was not Erin's story that impressed me as unique. What grabbed my heart was that an eight-year-old had *remembered* an abstract, second-hand story from a year earlier, because it was about long-term persistence and the power of prayer. God bless your prayers.

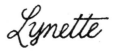

While enduring cancer and months of treatments, nearly all the cards, calls, food, and gifts I received were from Christians over the age of forty. Two exceptions to this were Leslie who gave me a prayer journal, and Wendy who immediately volunteered to cook a meal for us. Since she was rather new to our congregation, I did not even know her! Accompanying the meal Wendy made for us was a very sweet and lengthy letter. She explained that when she was sixteen years old, her mother had gone through breast cancer surgery and a hysterectomy at the same time. Today Wendy is a singular individual. We all need to teach our young people what it means to give that cup of cold water to the Lord and how to do that. Wendy's mother should be very proud that Wendy chose to take the trauma of her teenage years and have it bless people in far away times and places. I am certain that God is very pleased with Wendy's outreach.

During the time I was taking chemo treatments, a personal message that I especially liked came from Donna Habegger who wrote that as she drove her children to school, they would all pray for me. I knew that this was not only good for me, but it was also good for her children.

Each Wednesday evening in the girls' Bible class that I teach there is a ten-year-old named Chelsea who I see caring for three younger siblings. Chelsea happily participates in picking up the little ones after class, in being sure of their safety, and getting them to the bathroom. Her mother has discussed with her and exemplified to her the care of a friend who had cancer. These are investments in Chelsea's future here on earth and eternally. Each child needs to be shown how to be a care giver in a variety of ways and then expected to participate on whatever level he or she can.

Dear Nita,

Because you are the mother of school age children, I want to suggest something to help you give them hope. Envision hope. Draw a cartoon of hope, write a poem about it, or invent a mascot that embodies hope. You might even have your children buy you a stuffed animal and give it a spunky name. Take this mascot with you to the hospital or to each treatment. Tell the kids that this furry friend will remind you of them and all they mean to you. The toy can give them something tangibly positive that they are doing for you.

I have a grown son named Caleb. When he was about five years old, my mom made him a stuffed alligator that was about thirty inches long and had a huge mouth with jagged teeth made out of rick-rack. Caleb slept with Allie alligator every night. I asked him why he was never afraid of the alligator. He said that it was because Allie ate up his bad dreams. Years later, when Caleb's brother was about four, Caleb said, "Boone, I am going to give you Allie now, so that he can eat up your bad dreams." Nita, find your family its own version of Allie. Let it eat up their fears. It can become the embodiment of hope. Have your hope reach up to God, reach out to others, and reach within yourself.

Your Sister in Christ,

Lynette

Dr. Wendy Harpham, a mother of three young children, was an internist in private practice in Dallas when she was diagnosed with non-Hodgkin's lymphoma. During years of treatments and raising children, she has written *When a Parent Has Cancer: A Guide to Caring for Your Children*. She also authored a children's book called, *Becky and the Worry Cup*. Harpham wisely states that she chose to use the challenges of her illness to teach her children what she would have wanted them to learn if she had never been sick a day in her life. She warns that some children will not want to talk about illness, but advises the parent to insist that the child listen to the most basic facts to understand in general what is happening. Those basics might be, "Mom is sick, going to the hospital for a bone marrow transplant, and her hair will fall out because of the medicine to make her better." If your child does not want to know more, you tell him no more. If the child chooses to ask questions, then her questions will determine how much you tell her.

Medical upsets can sometimes make children regress. Therefore, if you have a child who was being rather independent, and now he has difficulty making decisions or going to sleep, or if grades begin to slip, do not be surprised. This is acceptable as long as it is discussed as temporary. When the child returns to dealing with his environments and associates in age appropriate ways, he is coping. However, if he gets stuck in a bad mood or a former stage of development, he has needs that are not being met. Give each child a safe place to express his fear or sadness. Conversations can help the child vent in a mature way and move forward. Dr. Harpham writes that regardless of how your child views your sickness and treatments, his perception of your illness will not be the same as yours. Accept that.

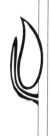

Give each child a safe place to express his fear or sadness.

When a parent has any sudden injury or illness, the old normal way of handling daily activities will not be the new normal. Trying to hold on to certain rigid roles and expectations can get frustrating and impossible. Be ready to adjust to fluctuating needs and abilities! For example, on days that immunity is low and the parent cannot be exposed to the children's germs, it is best that he or she keep her distance in order to maximize her chances of getting well.

While cancer changed many things in the life of Dr. Harpham and her children, she looks on it as only one part of their lives and does not let it define them. She asks that teachers and friends not repeat, "How's your mom," every time they see the children. Harpham wants her children to be able to escape the illness and to find moments when they can focus on just being kids. Give them chances to forget.

Five days before I began chemo treatments, I wrote a letter to my fifteen-year-old son. I had already talked to him about cancer and my struggles, but this letter was to give to him later when I was least myself.

Dear Boone,

This is to affirm to you that I love you dearly. I will still be loving you on days that I cannot hug you or mother you. I still love you when I am not myself. It is predicted that I will have various ailments and discomforts. Some will happen soon after treatments, and others will happen days or weeks later.

I am praying VERY specifically, and I want you to also. I know some very important people who are presidents of universities, owners of banks, and fancy lawyers, but with God their prayers have no more weight nor pull than yours. In fact, yours may be even more attention-grabbing to God, because yours are spoken with such love and with personal specifics. I know that God is more powerful than any problem, even cancer, chemo, hormones, or mental problems. Remember Shadrach, Meshach, and Abednego said, "Our God is able to deliver us, but even if He does not, we will serve only Him." It is scary to have so many unknowns. We are being called on to show that we can trust our loving Father God so much that we can feel secure in His love regardless of what is going on in our physical world. I am daily trying to cultivate this feeling. I do not want to be like the children of Israel as they stood at the edge of the Promised Land. Because of their fears, they believed the ten practical spies instead of Joshua and Caleb who faithfully ignored the physical evidence of powerful giants. Joshua and Caleb knew that God was more powerful than giants. I am standing at a new land; chemo, cancer, and the unknown are the giants I face. Listening to hymns and reading scriptures helps me. I do NOT feel let down by God, but I do get to feeling let down at myself when my fears seem bigger than my faith. That is why I especially value the faith of each person praying for me.

Satan and sin are the causes of sickness, and he can use it for temptation, as he did with Job. Satan has seen the adversity of sickness spiritually defeat many people, so he hopes to defeat millions more. We need to view this as a time of battle against the devil. But remember, God is more powerful than Satan, and God will not let us be burdened with more than we are capable of handling.

God's blessings to us are endless: a loving family, a loving church family, money to buy what we need, hospital insurance, good doctors not far from home, a washer and dryer, and many other assets.

Parts of Romans 8:18-37: For I consider that the sufferings of this present time are nothing to be compared with the glory that is to be revealed to us...We ourselves, having the first-fruits of the

Spirit, even we ourselves groan within ourselves, waiting eagerly for our adoption as sons, the redemption of our body. For in hope we have been saved, but hope that is seen is not hope; for why does one also hope for what he sees? But if we hope for what we do not see, with perseverance we wait eagerly for it. And in the same way, the Spirit also helps us with our weakness; for we do not know how to pray as we should, but the Spirit Himself intercedes for us with groanings too deep for words; and He who searches the hearts knows what the mind of the Spirit is, because He intercedes for the saints according to the will of God. And the will of God causes all things to work together for good to those who love God, to those who are called according to His purpose...Who shall separate us from the love of Christ? Shall tribulations, or distress, or persecution, or famine, or nakedness, or peril, or sword?...No, in all these things we overwhelmingly conquer through Him who loved us! (NAS)

I pray that we will come out of this much stronger spiritually and more able to help others!

Love,

Mom

My sons who were ages fifteen and twenty-two saw me in pain, frightened, confused, weak, extremely dependent, and unable to take care of them, but I was pleased that neither of them ignored my trials nor added to my problems. Each in his own ways was loving and helpful. Then they witnessed my spiritual focus sharpen. They realized I was discovering new meanings in many life experiences, scriptures, and songs. They saw both their dad and me get closer to God and closer to one another. As his response to my repeatedly saying that I was not brave, Boone said, "Mom, you are brave; you just don't know it!" Boone's statement told me that I had spent my life in spiritual preparation for these difficult times, but I would not know this bravery until I used it.

My older son Caleb lives 200 miles away, but he would work some extra time during the week so he could be with me longer on the weekends

I had been through chemo. Before my chemo began, he asked many questions of a friend whose mother had been through cancer a few years earlier. These trials gave us opportunities to have several heartfelt conversations. Caleb told me that he considered me a modern-day Job.

On a short-term basis, my husband had cared for me before, but my sons had not. I cherish ways the boys looked after me, the dialogues my cancer instigated, the new patience it induced, and priorities it readjusted.

For several months I wrote to Nita, a mother of children ages eleven to sixteen. She lives far away, and I had never met her. Unexpectedly she phoned saying she was accompanying her husband to Gatlinburg where he would speak at a retreat. I was thrilled to meet her there, especially after we turned out to be such kindred spirits. When I told her that her wig looked natural, she told me that most days she wears it, but occasionally she wears a baseball cap and the bald look, because she believes that occasionally healthy people need to face that.

Let your children see how to take care of sick people. By your example, they will learn physically helpful hints, and they will learn how to soothe those with aches or pains. In the 1980s when Boone was still a baby, one morning Morgan leaned over to change Boone's diaper and felt something pop. Morgan spent the day on the couch resting his hurting back muscles. After he had been flat on his back awhile, I brought him a drink. In order for him not to have to sit up, I put the liquid in a Tupperware sipper cup with the tall spout made for toddlers. I lifted Morgan's head and held the cup up to his mouth while our son Caleb watched and helped me, but when Caleb and I saw that big, hairy moustache hanging over the spout of the sipper cup, we started laughing.

for further
thought

for further thought

1. When should children be shielded from troubles such as job layoffs, poverty, alcoholism, divorce, sickness, and death, and when should they not?

2. How does age and maturity become important when deciding what to discuss with a child?

3. List ways to find out what is frightening to a child and design information and comforts specifically for him.

4. What is the possible peril of lying to a child?

5. Using Matthew 18:1-6, how do you think Christ wants us to be childlike but not childish? What are the positive connotations of one and the negative connotations of the other?

6. How can Godly faith be cultivated in a child who has prolonged sickness or who has a relative with illness?

7. Have all our children, whether sick or healthy, understood that Bible stories are about real people and not fictitious characters?

8. Are we as a family and as a church investing today in a soul-savings account for each child by storing up in his heart, mind, and soul precious Bible stories and specific verses that will sustain him when the future brings adversity? (Deuteronomy 6:6-9; Psalm 78:1-4; Psalm 119:105)

9. Explain the wisdom and comfort of Boone's statement, "Mom, you are brave; you just don't know it."

10. What messages do a person's example send a child who sees someone coping or not?

11. Describe additional ways that younger children might be encouraged to maintain hope using a calendar, learning new skills, getting rewards for accomplishments, or the heart warming thrill of helping someone else.

12. How did Barnabas' faith in young John Mark encourage him to not turn back on the next mission trip? (Acts 15:39) How did Barnabas' positive expectations probably help change John Mark? (II Timothy 4:11)

Chapter Eight

Grace, Prayer, and Comfort From Your History or Herstory

Songs

God Moves in a Mysterious Way

'Tis the Blessed Hour of Prayer

At Calvary (Years I Spent)

Amazing Grace

Take Time to Be Holy

Grace Greater Than Our Sin

What a Friend We Have in Jesus

Savior, Breathe an Evening Blessing

A Blessing in Prayer

Standing on the Promises

Sweet Hour of Prayer

Did You Think to Pray?

There's a Garden

His Grace Reaches Me

Wonderful Grace of Jesus

Awesome God, Guide me to **ultimate faith** in You in spite of the physical evidence of **my troubles**, helping me to learn, "Your grace is **sufficient**."

I have heard it said that one of the most difficult things to receive is grace. Not only is it difficult to explain, it is even difficult to fathom God's motivations to extend such lavish kindness to you and me. In addition, grace is many-faceted. Ponder what Jesus experienced in order to show us how to recognize grace and all it does. He was in heaven, surrounded by praise, perfection, joy, and comfort. He volunteered to experience: hunger, sprains, being hit, thirst, diarrhea, being sleep deprived, tears, tooth decay, vomiting, backaches, blisters, bug bites, diseases, cuts, sore throats, headaches, thorns, and nails. Why did Jesus spend thirty-three years on earth? Why not just come to earth, spend a few days, and die for our sins? Because He wanted us to trust Him and believe Him—therefore, He tried to SHOW us grace, not only in what He gave up for us, but also by what He endured and understood first-hand. Hebrews 4:15 tells us that Jesus was tempted just like us in every way. That means that He struggled like us. As Dr. John Mark Hicks says, "Jesus was not Teflon-Man with temptations bouncing off of Him. He struggled." Jesus prayed, "Father, if it is possible, may this cup be taken from me."

Jesus saw the future. Yet, He volunteered to suffer the agony of dread, be grabbed by fear in the night, be tortured by people, whips, and spikes, and then be tormented by our sins. Barbara Johnson writes that GRACE stands for **G**od's **R**iches **A**t **C**hrist's **E**xpense. If you and I could fully comprehend how deeply and personally we are loved by God, we would not be so mystified by grace, nor would we thwart it so. It is God's grace that saves us, but we must grab it just like a drowning man would reach for the life preserver thrown to him. The drowning man does not save himself; it is the one who threw the life preserver and the lifesaver itself that saves the man. Our assignment is not to decipher every divine mystery, but to ask, seek, and knock, following God's Word and feeding our faith in the one who is called Providence—the One who creates, sustains, ordains, maintains, and loves.

Dear Kay,

I made a salad for supper and wish we lived close enough that I could give you half. During my most difficult times, I longed for a closeness to God. I have grown up very blessed, so I feel He expects a lot of me. God is perfect. I've let Him down by being timid to tell people about Him, being envious, wanting revenge, being resentful, prideful, or judgmental. My guilty feelings distance me from God. There are religious groups that place top priority on performance, works, and guilt. Other groups of religious people believe that once you are saved, you are always saved, regardless of what you do. God's Truth as revealed in the New Testament lies between these two extremes. Cancer has caused me to do more praying, scripture reading, and contemplating grace, thus slowly improving my relationship with Him.

In school or at work, we are used to a system that gives rewards for good performances and punishment for bad actions. Jesus emphasizes the love of God and responding love which causes the person to improve his performances. The Lord's story of two brothers answers many questions about performance and forgiveness. Bill Watkins has a wonderful sermon on this parable. This is not the story of one person in God's family and one outside God's family. They are brothers with the same father. The older son follows the rules. The younger boy breaks social standards, moral codes, and religious laws. He is probably gone a very long time. Yet when he returns, he finds his dad still patiently awaiting and even running to met him, not because of the boy's performance, but because it is the father's loving nature. It was undignified for a Jewish patriarch to run, but the father runs to meet his son, in spite of protocol. The father sees the boy's needs and loves filling them. He still hates sin, because it is so bad on the boy, but he deeply loves the sinner. The boy focuses attention on his sin. As the father tries to do loving things for him, the boy reminds the dad of those sins. Nevertheless, the father tells servants to bring the best robe, ring, and sandals, and throw a party. The robe clothes him and tells his status. The ring is probably a signet ring that announces to what family he belongs. At baptism, God dresses us with the blood of Jesus; it continues to mark our hearts, tells our status, and proclaims that we belong to the family of God. Neither son is loved more or less because of his performance. Recognizing God's love and grace causes us to work on our performances.

Several of Jesus' listeners became angry or confused as Jesus talked like this. At other times Jesus told the eternal dangers of calling someone a fool or lusting in your heart. When even thoughts can condemn us, who's good enough for God? No one. That is the point! We each need Jesus' blood to continue covering our sins and marking our hearts.

What a relief to embrace the truth about grace and stop "getting the cart before the horse." When we admit with our hearts, minds, and souls that our performances will never measure up to God's standards, then we can stop trying to make it on our own, and instead concentrate on our childlike relationship with Him. My life becomes a response of thanks.

As our minister, David Jackson says, "Live your love!"

Love,

Lynette

Prayer is a circular driveway that makes it possible for us to, "ask, seek, knock," acknowledge our needs and God's power, be open to His answers, thank Him, and start the process all over again.

Dear Nancy,

It was during my darkest days that I truly began to see with the eyes of my heart the meaning of the phrase, "I covet your prayers." I had heard this phrase in my younger days. I don't remember hearing it in the last decade or two. I knew that I needed the prayers of every person who had ever known me and needed the prayers of any Christian willing to pray for me. We share the bond of Christ. Prayer lets you know you have once again been put at the center of God's attention but each time by a different intercessor. Each person who recruits others to pray for you shows his love for you, his faith, his sympathy, and trust in the results. Even though God is taking care of millions of other individuals, you were not put on a waiting list. He cares for you better than a hen with one chick.

Genesis 18:14 "Is anything too difficult for the Lord?" (NAS)

Praying for you daily,

Lynette

Dear Lillard,

I hope you are still finding comfort in envisioning individuals and classes praying for you. Some Christian speakers insist that God does not care about the details of our lives. They assume that we should mush our way through certain issues on our own and then assign some arbitrary point as the line of demarcation between small problems and big problems. God should only be bothered with big problems, since in their opinions to bother God with our minutia is to trivialize His greatness. In contrast, this is how I look at it. My fifteen-year-old son Boone tells me many things in which I have NO interest; however, because he is my child, I find all he says precious, not because of the subject but because of my love for the speaker. Often I hear about the P-38J Lightning and the P-51D Mustang. I could not care less about these World War II fighter planes. However, I know that Boone's telling me about his interests, joys, fears, and needs shows that he wants a real relationship with me. I am glad Boone does not edit his conversations with me or hold back from discussing things with me until he deems them important enough. God has much deeper and more perfect love for us than we do for our children. Therefore, I believe He truly wants us to take Him at His word and not only "cast all our cares on Him," but also share with Him all the emotions and details a child would share with a loving parent.

Yours Truly,

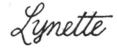

Dear John,

As you know, our house is surrounded by woods. Often as we drive down the road, a turtle, deer, or squirrel will run out in front of our car. Each continues on its way, except the squirrels. Cars are trauma in their lives. After all, the squirrel has started across a path in his territory when a car monster heads toward him. So, first he continues, then he decides it would be better to turn back, next he goes right, dashes left, abruptly stops, ponders, and finally does what he intended to do in the first place. Morgan has tried to anticipate what a squirrel will do, but it's useless and aggravating. Morgan asks why squirrels keep repeating this stupid panic behavior. I identify greatly with each squirrel. A trauma comes into my life, but I continue looking to God, next I get very fearful, then I get calm, suddenly I panic, I compose myself with encouraging scriptures, but then I imagine the worst. I pray but become distracted by worry, I feel all alone and uncared for, and finally, I get back to faith in God and make it across the road—through the trauma. I hope I learn my lessons better than the squirrels. The next time you hear someone called "squirrelly," remember my story and smile.

Sincerely,

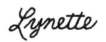

Years ago, I heard the story of a little girl who became afraid during a storm. The child's mother had put her to bed, but as lightening flashed and thunder clapped and then rumbled, the child called her mother back. In a frightened voice, the girl told her mama she wanted someone to stay with her during the storm. The mother reminded her little one that God is always with us. To that, the girl replied, "Well, I want someone with skin on!" Sometimes we all want someone with "skin on" to be with us in the flesh or at least in our mind's eye. Of course, Jesus came and lived as a human to show us that He could also have "skin on." However, since we have never really seen Him physically, or even a picture of Him, it is difficult to imagine how He would look. Therefore, besides the comforts you can receive from scriptures, songs, prayers, cards, letters, and the voices of friends, I encourage you to look into your own past for a different type of comfort and strength.

Dear Beverly,

The cancer diagnosis made me long for strength, bravery, and wisdom. Learning about cancer's treatments made me yearn for those traits even more. Often I prayed that I would discern what lessons God wanted me to cull out of these circumstances.

My friend Rosemary told me that when she wonders how she will handle a frightening situation, she thinks of her grandmother. Near the beginning of the 1900s, a sixteen-year-old girl left Europe all alone to cross the Atlantic in the steerage of a ship. This young lady later became Rosemary's grandmother. Rosemary has felt empowered by knowing that if her inexperienced future grandmother could be so brave, strong, and smart, Rosemary herself could also. If there are stories of strength and endurance among your ancestors, use them to bolster your own resolve. If you ponder this idea, you may even rediscover stories in your own past when you yourself were bolder, stronger, or wiser than you had previously known.

As a child, I heard many Bible lessons with facts about specific Bible characters. I received these from: my parents, my Bible classes, the pulpit, my school, the songs I sang, and from my Bible story books with the beautiful pictures which I scrutinized. When I matured and was told that the people in these stories were Jews, but I was not, I remember feeling I had lost a connection to them which I had falsely thought I possessed. Later, I learned that the connection which I had felt as a little child was really true but in a different way. Joseph, Jocabed, Miriam, Hannah, and the Shunammite woman who built the room for Elisha were my favorites. Christians are connected to them spiritually because of Jesus Christ, His death, resurrection, and our semblance of that in baptism. I love the song that says, "Father Abraham had many sons; many sons had father Abraham. I am one of them and so are you, so let's all praise the Lord." In the same ways we use stories of our physical ancestors, also use stories of your spiritual ancestors. Struggles of contemporary Christians can also help you. Using forebearers, spiritual ancestors, or fellow Christians can each be another facet of asking God to put the right people, the correct information, and the best advice into your life.

Praying for you,

Lynette

Dear Edd,

Now is a time to look to stories from your own family's past for lessons of your ancestors who have endured through difficult times. Use both physical and spiritual ancestors to give you strength so that like them, you can persevere.

As I underwent surgery and began chemo, I wondered what my grandmother would have told me if she were alive today. While she was still living, I had no health traumas, so I cannot call up any such advice from her. What I can use as her advice is the way she lived her life constantly adapting and never acting as if life had cheated her or owed her more.

Deedie Slate lived in Macon County, Tennessee near Lafayette. One would be hard pressed to find an area with fewer economic opportunities. Their school went only to the eighth grade, but her "Pappy," knowing the value of an education, worked extra hard so that after her eighth grade year he could send Deedie to a private academy for a couple of years. Eventually, she married Hova Carnahan and had three children. Deedie also helped raise a niece whose mama had died. When Lewis, her oldest, was fifteen, a spark from the chimney caught the roof on fire. Hova went up on the roof to fight the fire. He caught pneumonia and died. Now Deedie was left with no husband, no house, and three children to support. She had no car and could not drive. Deedie took a job in the school cafeteria and became its manager. Each morning as the bus came by for the children, she would ride to school with them. In three more years her son Lewis graduated from high school.

Then in the midst of World War II, the army called Lewis, and Deedie worried that he would be killed.

As the army transported Lewis from one place to another, Deedie fervently prayed. All his company was sent to fight in the Pacific. However, Lewis' papers were lost, so he could not be sent. He became a medic in Missouri. Oh, the power of this mother's prayers! When Lewis returned from the army, he enrolled at David Lipscomb College in Nashville. Therefore, Deedie adapted and moved herself and her two daughters to Nashville also. Lewis graduated, found a wife, managed a store, and became a father. Then because of a faulty furnace, Deedie's Nashville house also burned to the ground.

How does a woman who cannot drive adapt and make money? Deedie bought a duplex that was near enough to the church building and the grocery store to walk. She lived in one side of the duplex and rented out the other side. During weekdays, she kept children and baby sat for others on the weekends. She took in ironing and sold greeting cards. She investigated applicants from the Nashville Diesel School who were from Macon County. If their backgrounds checked out, she took in the young men as boarders in her tiny upstairs room. Deedie continued to pay into Social Security so she would have ten years of contributing in order to later receive Social Security. Then Deedie had to keep going to the doctor with a cough that worsened. She had tuberculosis, but she adapted to living at the TB Hospital. Deedie conquered that also and returned to her regular way of life. Through it all, she rarely complained. I have never known a woman who did such lowly jobs yet earned so much honor among those who knew her.

Daily she read her Bible. She knew what it said and lived by it. She sang hymns as she worked. For decades she fought arthritis that gnarled her hands and feet. Eventually, she had to live in an assisted living facility. She continued to adapt. After being there a few years, she was sent to a hospital for a few days. Because of the hospital's poor treatment, Deedie was burned and had to go through painful procedures and eventually have her leg amputated. She adapted again. This time it was as an elderly woman learning how to lift herself out of the bed into a wheelchair, getting herself around Heartland's three-story building, and functioning on her own. Whenever we went to see her, her face lit up. Instead of bending our ears looking for sympathy, she focused on asking about the grandchildren or the great grandchildren. Grandmother had high expectations for each of us, and she prioritized the spiritual expectations as the most paramount. This humble woman from the land of little opportunity, dogged by tragedy and trauma, is still influencing people. She has mothered and meekly mentored future ministers, elders, and teachers.

As I look to Grandmother most of all for being a Christian woman who graciously adapted, can I look at my troubles and do any less? I want to some day be together with her in heaven and for Jesus to say, "I see the spiritual resemblances, and I am proud of you both."

Your Sister in Christ,

Lynette

Dear Janie Ruth,

Last month we had a storm with high winds. After it was over, as we drove down our road which is lined with woods, I saw a couple of trees had fallen. Among thousands of trees, why had those fallen while others stood? I thought of people blown by the high winds of trauma. Why do some people collapse spiritually as they undergo extended sickness? Why do others mature and become enriched and bless the lives of those around them? Much of our life here on earth is spent grasping at shadows. Sickness can show a person what is the real substance and what is shadow. Aesop tells the story of a dog with a bone in his mouth who sees his reflection in water. Thinking the reflection is another dog with a bigger bone, he opens his mouth to grab the reflection and loses his bone. The moral is: Beware that you do not lose the substance by grasping at the shadow.

II Corinthians 4:16-18 (paraphrased): Don't give up; even though our bodies are gradually decaying, our inner person is being strengthened and renewed each day. These troubles which are really so temporary, are getting us ready for a permanent, glorious and solid reward far out of proportion to all our pain, because we are concentrating on things that are invisible, not what we see. For visible things are here for a little while and then gone, but it is invisible things that are really permanent.

God Bless You,

Dear Nita,

In 1993, we had a blizzard and no electricity for six days. On the morning we awoke to snow eighteen inches deep, my husband Morgan walked down our steep hill to survey the road. Neighbors told him the house near us, which had been vacant, was about to have new inhabitants, and they might have already come. Morgan high-stepped his way over and knocked on the door. He met the two who had moved in the day before. They had hardly any food and were snuggled in the bed trying to stay warm. Surrounded by their five acres of woods, they had no dry firewood. Plus, when our area has no electricity, we have no water, because our wells require electric pumps. Morgan told the new couple, Pat and Bob, to come stay with us.

We thanked God for our wood burning stove and all the supplies we had stored, from flashlights and batteries to food and water. We had a fire perpetually going in the wood burning stove. We scooped up snow to melt so we could wash dishes and melted extra snow to pour in the commode so that it would flush. Pat and Bob brought an iron pot with a lid. We used it and my ironware to cook. We put bricks in the fire's coals to set a Pyrex dish of food on. We took food out of our now incapacitated refrigerator and stored the provisions in the snow.

Because snow came up higher than a vehicle's axle, no car or truck could leave our road, and no county crew would come scrape. Morgan and neighborhood men shoveled a path out. With snow being eighteen inches deep and the road being one and a half miles of hills and curves, that took hours. However, when a path was cleared, some families left to live with relatives. I was proud that I endured like a pioneer, cooking over an open fire, taking care of a family of four, and for forty hours had guests whom we had previously never even met.

In the same ways that we survived the blizzard, seven years later I survived chemo: (1) We prayed. (2) I used resources (physical, mental, and spiritual) that I had in storage. (3) I used creative solutions to some problems. (4) We pooled our resources with those of others. (5) I welcomed help. (6) I made my way through one task at a time, not knowing when the trial would be over. (7) At the end, I was proud that I had coped, learned, and had not given up.

Nita, there may be an experience in your own past that you can use to help you relearn to cope. Decide which exact resources you need, which ones you have, which ones you can ask other people for, and which ones you need to rely on God to give you. From one pioneer to another, I send my best wishes and daily prayers,

Lynette

Dear Sharon,

There are many things I repeat to myself. This is comparable to Deuteronomy 6 where God tells fathers to explain to their children about God and His commands, as the family sits in the house, walks, goes to bed, and gets up. God says to "tie them on your finger, put them on your forehead, and write them on your doorposts." God knows we humans need perpetual reminders of Him.

A few days ago, I was reading Hebrews 11—12:2 "Therefore, since we have so great a cloud of witnesses surrounding us, let us lay aside every encumbrance, and the sin which so easily entangles us, and let us run with endurance the race that is set before us, fixing our eyes on Jesus, the Author and Perfecter of our faith, who for the joy set before Him endured the cross, despising the shame, and has set down at the right hand of the throne of God." (NAS)

These witnesses testify that God rewards us, loves us, and is unchanging. However, this makes me think of the fact that people going through struggles can best be cheered on and most believably comforted by others who have gone through similar troubles. The men and women of Hebrews 11 are our "great cloud of witnesses." They show us that faith is much more than mental. Faith causes actions to happen, both on the part of the humans and on the part of God. It is informative to read Hebrews 11 and list every verb that was initiated by faith.

At the Olympics, almost none of the people in the stands has endured what the current participants are going though in training, pain, challenges, blows, and battles. However, similarly to us, many of our "great cloud of witnesses" have been through disease, disappointments, repeated losses of earthly security, attacks on their faith, physical pain, fearfulness, struggling with which decision to make, crummy remarks, and mental anguish. And, while enduring all this, Job also suffered the disastrous death of all his ten children on the same day. Friends said Job was to blame for his own problems!

Noah, Sarah, and many others are also in the stands cheering for you. Rely on them. Use the examples of their *failings* to give you hope—hope because this shows that God loves us even though we have been weak, made wrong assumptions, doubted Him, and not reached out to others. Use the examples of their *faithfulness* to give you hope—hope because it proves that God can help us become stronger, help us understand Him more deeply, see His compassion and majesty, and reach out to others. Do I think that every one listed in Faith's Hall of Fame knew that he or she was a great example of faith who would be speaking to us thousands of years later? I think not! That gives me sweet comfort to see that God does not expect super-human faith to be our constant frame of mind; He expects us to feed our faith and use our struggles to let Him continually grow our faith. Eventually, like the faithful who have gone before us, even while still on this earth, we will be able to feel a spiritual realm that is beyond the reality of our five senses and lifts us to new faithfulness, only because we have gone through these present hardships.

May God open your eyes to see more blessings and opportunities and open your ears to hear more spiritual music and meaning. May He have you touched by more hugs and tasting the wonderful foods that Christian friends have made for you.

God Bless You,

Lynette

for further thought

1. What is the difference between mercy and grace?
2. What does the story of the lost boy in Luke 15 tell us about God's grace?
3. Was Christ's coming to earth to die for us a later after-thought? (John 1:1-5; Ephesians 1:3-12)
4. Did He sweat, bleed, cry, dread, and hurt like we do? (Isaiah 53:4-7; Luke 22:39-45; Philippians 2:5-8)
5. On the cross, what besides the nails, thorns, and mockery put Jesus through agony? (Isaiah 53:10-12)
6. How does trying to earn our own salvation show we are "putting the cart before the horse?"
7. Does casting all our cares on God include telling Him details?
8. Think of a time when you have acted "squirrelly." Explain how spiritual focus helps us not act "squirrelly."
9. Is the statement true or false that the more we appreciate what Jesus did for us, the more appropriate our responses to Him will be? (Ephesians 2:8-10)
10. From which of your ancestors can you draw courage? Why?
11. What Bible character's life is your favorite example? Are you helped by both his failings and his faithfulness?
12. Name an adventure or a trauma that happened in your life in which you were pleased with how you coped.

Chapter Nine
"Miserable Comforters"
What the Sick Need and What They Do Not

Songs

O Love That Will Not Let Me Go

Each Day I'll Do (Beautiful Life)

Where Could I Go But to the Lord?

God's Wonderful People

The Lord Bless You and Keep You

Brighten the Corner Where You Are

I Have a Savior (For You I Am Praying)

To Love Someone More Dearly Every Day

God Bless You, Go With God

A Common Love

Freely, Freely

God Be With You

Let the Words of My Mouth

Take My Life and Let It Be

God, as You are Perfect Love and I want to be like You, help me to love the messenger and focus on his or her care for me even if his message is not always a comfort.

Chemotherapy is a unique experience. One book I read said there are forty different types of chemo, while another said there are eighty types. Regardless, most people do not know much about these. It seems to me that every person who spoke of chemo in the life of one of his or her family members told me what happened to his loved one as if the exact same thing would certainly happen to me. Do not expect certain side-effects; wait to see what happens. Plus, treatments are constantly being improved.

Dear Susan,

Books and brochures I had been given regarding chemo terrified me. I hated to even look inside the chemo room. I would like to explain the process in non-medical terms, giving you enough knowledge to feel that you can handle it. Some procedures vary from one doctor's office to the next, but other ways of doing things are the same at each clinic.

It cannot be over emphasized that no two people will have exactly the same side-effects to chemo, even if they are on the same drugs. Twenty-four hours before you are to go to chemo, pour water into a glass, then pour that water into a pitcher. Do this eight times, and throughout the day, drink it all. By the next day, when you have the blood test and chemo, your vein will be easier to find, and your kidneys will be better ready to face the drugs. Also, remember to be warm, have your arm warm, exercise prior to the test, and avoid caffeine.

Oncology nurses I had were special people, sometimes assertive, but caring and attentive. Ask the nurse questions. Tell her what bothers you, and bond with her in every way you can. With each oncology nurse, I told her or him, "I do not want to SEE what is done, so I will be turning my head." If the nurse began talking to another patient about something I did not want to hear, I put on earphones with CDs of hymns. If you start feeling weird in any way, tell your nurse. The IV drip can be slowed, and sometimes your symptoms will go away.

Before each treatment is a blood test to tell if blood counts are healthy enough to receive chemo. Then I was given something in the IV to hydrate me and a drug to relax me. I felt my eyes get big, it gave me a sudden happy thrill and then I was a little calmer. Next, I was given one anti-nausea drug and then another. That makes four different fluids given individually before the chemo started. Drugs were never combined in the drip. Then one chemo drug was put in and followed by the other. Finally, I would get something to rinse out my veins. Waiting at home was an already-filled prescription of anti-nausea pills. Some of them made me sleepy, and that was a good thing. Sleep was my friend. You can make it; this wimp did.

Sincerely,

Lynette

My husband and sons were the only people who saw what chemo did to me. Regardless, I had some loving people who kept saying if I kept a good attitude, side-effects would be minimal. None of these "advisors" had been through chemo themselves. Some aspects of my chemo were exactly like the majority of patients, but I had other reactions that were unique and unlike experiences predicted in books. No one can guess which of your experiences will be usual and which will be exceptional. Before the process, I did not know enough to ask many specific questions. Plus, information I had been given regarding what to expect greatly frightened me. Warnings of all that could possibly go wrong gave me negative information overload. In the place of conceivable disasters, I needed to hear helpful hints to get organized for the cancer struggle, medical strategies to make the coping easier, psychological tactics to soothe my worries, and spiritual reassurances about depending on God. Because at the first round of chemo I was such a complete novice and because drugs can blur one's mind, memory, and inner clock, it was very advisable to write down each drug taken, when it was taken, and any side-effects. Later, I took this information to my oncologist, asking if all had gone the way it was expected to go.

In the book of Job, when Eliphaz, Bildad, and Zophar come to console Job, for the first seven days they are silent. That is probably their best time with him. All sufferers need to be heard whether they are speaking in words or tears. Listen graciously without butting in or changing the subject. Let the sufferer decide the subject and set the pace. Avoid saying, "I know how you feel," or telling the sufferer how he is "supposed" to feel. Later, Eliphaz, Bildad, and Zophar begin telling Job that God blesses those who obey Him, therefore, Job's suffering proves that he has not obeyed God. Yes, God does bless those who obey Him, but the blessing may not be what we thought it would be. Even when we suffer and ask questions, God can still be blessing us. Even though part of what Eliphaz, Bildad, and Zophar say is true, part is not true, and it becomes a great aggravation to Job. I find it remarkable that this ancient man Job invented the oxymoron, "miserable comforters" (Job 16:2). In order to *not* be a miserable comforter yourself, do not assume you can prophesy what will

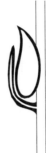

Even when we suffer and ask questions, God can still be blessing us.

happen while on chemo. If it is your friend or family member going through chemo, speak of your prayers for him, your love for her, and the power and love of God even when times are difficult. Keep in mind that there are events in life that God did not cause, but He can use for good even though they are not "good" in our definition of that word. If it is a death, a divorce, or being fired that plagues your friend, do not say that it was God's will. It is a gigantic understatement to say life is complicated. Since when has God made any of us privy to his exact M.O. in any specific event? Even if He explained it, we could not understand.

Someone close to me works in the field of medicine. He is very well educated, experienced, and keeps knowledgeable concerning the latest in cancer medicines. However, as the year 2000 was ending, he was not yet sympathetically wise. He stated, "If you keep a good attitude, you won't throw up. The only people on chemo who throw up are those who expect to." Then he convinced others of his expertise in how my body should react. Next, two individuals with whom he had spoken called me with pep talks for the power of a good attitude. This became a great burden to me. Trying to advise me, these three became my Eliphaz, Bildad, and Zophar. Like Job's miserable comforters, part of what they said was true, but part was not. It is true that anti-nausea drugs are wonderful, but that does not negate the fact that each person is an individual. It is true that an optimistic attitude can help, but do not lay extra burdens on the patient, insisting that her attitude will determine chemo's severity! Later, I thought of a video that I had seen about a doctor who was doing exactly what physicians are trained to do—being smart, current, and efficient in their specialties. Yet, this doctor in the movie was not compassionate. Yes, he had *seen* the things that happen to cancer patients, but he had not opened the eyes of his heart. Then in the movie, the doctor himself gets cancer, and everything changes drastically. He learns to listen to his patients with the ears and heart of experience, understands his patients as unique individuals, and tries to find solutions. The doctor changes from being a competent doctor and crummy person to become a compassionate person who is also an outstanding doctor. There is a vast difference between knowledge and wisdom.

"I'm certain everything will turn our fine," was the statement that greatly aggravated one woman going through a double mastectomy, removal of lymph nodes, and chemo. Of course, her friends did not know the future, therefore their proclamation became a burden to my friend. Such a statement actually tells more about what the speaker is not willing to face than what he or she really knows. We have deep faith in what our God is capable of, but we do not know what His specific time-table and reasoning are. *Even struggles that can abundantly bless us eternally may be beyond our understanding in the present.* Predicting an exact medical outcome would be having the gift of prophecy. In Genesis 32, God changes Jacob's name to Israel because he has struggled with God. Being now the spiritual Israel, we as seekers sometimes "struggle" with God by asking questions. In contrast, the faithless do not wrestle. Reassurances to strugglers that are most comforting and valid include such statements as: I hate that this happened to you; there are many things we cannot understand on this side of eternity; I love you; God listens to every word you pray and is sustaining you in ways we cannot fathom; fellow Christians are imploring God on your behalf; God has a history of turning bad into good; and God has a

> **Even struggles that can abundantly bless us eternally may be beyond our understanding in the present.**

history of empowering the weak, the frightened, and the needy to become mighty victors.

As soon as my friend Ray heard that I had cancer, he came up to me and said, "I have a lot of questions to ask God!" This wise servant of God was telling me he did not really understand why God would let me suffer. I treasure his response, not as weak faith or lack of knowledge but as brimming with compassion.

Dear Melba,

I have a friend named Becky. She both tells and shows others the attitudes and actions of Jesus. When it was discovered that Becky had cancer, she seemed to know how to take good care of herself. Later, when I had chemo, I told Becky some people with good intentions had been my "Eliphaz, Bildad, and Zophar" by insisting that a really optimistic attitude would make chemo side-effects minimal. Their philosophy made me feel trapped. Becky said a chemo nurse preached to her the philosophy of "pull yourself up by your own bootstraps." The nurse told Becky that if she would just keep a perky attitude, chemo effects would be minimal. Becky sweetly said, "I do not appreciate that attitude; it implies that people who do not make it through their fight with cancer have only themselves to blame."

"Way to go Becky!" I thought. Later, Becky went to a dentist who specializes in gums. The dentist had an assistant who blathered on about her grandmother dying of breast cancer. Becky changed dentists! She was determined to not have negativity in her life in any form, even if it came disguised as spunkiness. Now that her treatments are over, Becky tells doctors she will not give blood samples at every "drop of the hat." They can take blood once, get all they want, divide it, and then not bother her arm. Becky may sound bossy, but she really is not. There are many ways in which she is my hero. Now, Becky and her husband have Bible study classes in their home. She reaches out to others. She initiated the call to uplift me.

If you have any such "miserable comforters," remember that perhaps unknowingly their message was as much sent by Satan as the fatal wind, the loss of income, and the pain of sores that were sent to Job. After all, Satan does use half-truths to hit us with when we are down. He did this to Jesus in the wilderness. (Matthew 4) However, God has much more power and wants you to tell Him your specific needs, not thinking you are strong enough to handle problems on your own. Lean on those Everlasting Arms that want to sweetly cradle you.

You are not alone.

Lynette

Dear Diane,

I pray that you are finding comforts from without and within. Make the most of them.

For several years the Bible class I have taught has been girls ages eight to eleven. I design my own teaching materials based on areas of the Bible which most curriculum does not cover in detail. Several years ago, before I had cancer, I had a student named Lydia who requested that I teach a unit on Job. So now with each new collection of girls, I once again teach lessons on Job. I spend weeks drilling them on facts, hearing them say memory verses, discussing the concept of faithful perseverance, and acting out modern applications. Since eight-year-olds do not understand the meaning of an oxymoron, last week I endeavored to act out "miserable comforters." I stood mimicking an agonizing face, an afflicted posture, and tortured limbs, then used a deep, tormented voice to say the word "miserable." Immediately, in a gentle, sweetly consoling voice with demeanor that suggested the relief of a soothing bath, I sang "comforters." I quickly performed this contrast several times and then asked them what Job's nickname for Eliphaz, Bildad, and Zophar meant. They each wanted to be the one to first solve the challenge, but as they grappled with how to articulate the interpretation, Erin said, "It means hurting help." "Exactly!" I exclaimed. We went on to discuss how someone could come to help a sufferer but in the process say things that could be a burden. At this point, Whitney wanted me to explain what a burden is.

I told athletic, rambunctious Whitney to walk from the wall to the chair in the middle of the room. She easily did so. Then I told her to come back to the wall and do it again. This time as Whitney tried to walk those eight feet, I held her shoulders, so she had to drag me with her. When she arrived at the chair, I said, "That is what it means to have a burden." She exalted in having been victorious even though she was weighed down by a burden. Not only did the class have a new image in their minds to help them remember the meaning of "miserable comforters" and "burden," it led them into a discussion of specific sentiments we each should say or not say when someone suffers with illness, grief, or disaster.

I proceeded to untangle the idea that remarks made by some comforters are partially true and partially false. The Eliphaz group told Job that God blesses those who follow Him. I asked my class if this is true. They knew that it is. Then Job's friends proclaimed that since God blesses those who follow Him, Job's severe suffering must mean his life was full of horrible sinning. My students saw this was not true because God had delighted in Job's behavior.

Next, I told of when I dreaded chemo beginning and experienced my own "miserable comforters." Assuming that my class' answers would be words such as "sad" or "burdened," I explained how three people who loved me had insisted that a good attitude would make me not vomit or be nauseous, and then I asked the girls, "How do you think this remark made me feel?" "Nauseous!" said Whitney. I burst out laughing! I knew that in spite of her young age, Whitney had gained many lessons that night. She really understood the need for specific sympathy tempered with total truth. May you Diane also find such comforts from within and without. Sometimes they may even come form the heart and mouth of a child.

Love,

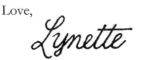

145

Becky and I were advised to "pull ourselves up by our bootstraps." In contrast, God said, "Cast all your cares on me." He wants us to tell Him our needs, not thinking we are mighty enough to handle life with a perky attitude. I also find it discomforting when people tell us God does not care about those details of our lives. They advise that we take care of the details and leave weightier matters to God. If God does not care about details, why did He create gorgeous colors, give us delicious foods, instill songs in birds, and dust butterflies with iridescence? He could have made the world with no color, no fragrance, no taste, no songs, and identical textures; we would have never known the difference! But, God INVENTED DETAILS! He instills in each honeybee a dance of communication. He clothes the lily and cares for the sparrow. He knows the number of hairs on each person's head; that is details.

Dear Lavonne,

Mattie Lou told me of your cancer. Recently, I too have been through a fight with cancer and all the uncertainty Satan tries to emphasize in our lives. I hope you are envisioning yourself being tenderly held in God's arms. To pray about any detail of your life that gives you fear or pain is not selfish; it is wise dependence on the Heavenly Father.

Take good care of yourself. Look for resources, not reprimands. Each current day will have enough to deal with, so do not transport any haunts from the past or possibilities from the future. Cull out only sweet memories and pretty panoramas.

It is good when others can help give you the resources you need: information, care, food, prayer, transportation, or encouragement. However, do not let others assign you the feelings they believe you should have right now. Some people may believe that you should be angry. Other individuals will want to stress a perky attitude. One woman insisted that I should make myself have feelings that were more "effective." Instead of being burdened by the assignments of feelings that other people say you should have, go to God. Let Him help shape your feelings. Prayer can help you see how dependent you are. Use your own words, phrases, and idioms to frame your requests and appreciations in the deep humility of dependence. If you are having trouble getting deep enough into your prayers, pray for more ability to pray. I am sure that reading scriptures has also helped you improve your prayers.

Let your *intellect* help you see the purposes of prayer by studying various psalms and their content. Let your *ears* help you hear the importance of prayer by speaking some of your supplications aloud. Let your *time* help you see the importance of prayer by increasing the minutes you devote to communication with God. Let your *body* sometimes help you speak your prayers through bowing, kneeling, or with tears. Let your *hands* help you see the importance of prayer by writing down some of your own petitions.

Once I heard a nervous young lawyer lead a public prayer. He began his appeal with, "Your Honor...." I don't think he meant to begin this way, but I thought, "How very appropriate!" Besides the fact that it was reverent, he had used his own words. Even if the words came by accident, they put us in mind of the fact that God is the Divine Judge and worthy of reverence. Most of all, I admired that they were uniquely personal.

I pray daily for you. May God bless your prayers and show you His answers,

Lynette

A few well-meaning people told me about every wreck and disaster they had recently seen or that had been in the news. At that time, I did not need to hear of such events; it made the world seem too hopeless. A couple of lovely ladies gave me books that I found miserable comfort. Two books said that it was certain that anyone who had enough faith would assuredly have her health made new. If her health was not restored, then it was because she did not have enough faith. In contrast, from the example of the apostle Paul and his "thorn in the flesh," we see that the believer does not always receive what he asks of the Lord. In II Corinthians 12, God tells Paul, "My grace is sufficient for you, for My strength is made perfect in weakness." (NKJV) God would not take away whatever was Paul's chronic ailment. Another book I was given was about "healing crystals" and New Age strategies. Be sure any book you give is truly comforting.

While I was still under the effects of chemo, I had people asking if my hair had grown back yet. Discuss hair only if the bald person brings up that subject. A few oncology nurses apply cooling caps so patients will not lose their hair. My investigations tell me that this is not wise, since it hampers the flow of chemo drugs to that area. Even though it was difficult to be bald, after being touched by a life-threatening disease, the loss of one's hair is far down on the list of real priorities.

Dear Sue,

Look for God's comfort specifically to you from whatever person, scripture, song, gift, or story that comes to you. It may come from a place you would have never predicted, from a person you would have never expected, or in ways that can thrill you. Do not be embarrassed to receive food. It may be difficult to be on the receiving end of this, but learn to let people give to you so that they can show their love for you and for God.

Your Sister in Christ,

While I was on chemo, Morgan and I learned some things by trial and error concerning how to care for me. God blessed us with a few good ideas I tell you so you can possibly use the ideas and not feel alone.

Dear Susan,

I wanted to tell you the reasons I wrote down each medicine that I took and my reactions. At first I just scribbled them down in my spiral notebook. Later I typed them, so I would have a copy to give to the oncologist to ask if I was reacting as expected. My mind might be too foggy to remember when what had happened. If something out of the ordinary developed, I could look back at my timetable and figure out the cause. The doctor could make a substitution. The day I was given chemo treatments was called Day 1 and all days of each cycle were numbered. On subsequent cycles if my eyes hurt on Day 15, I could look back at the previous Day 15. Seeing when it went away gave me hope.

In Christian Love,

Lynette

Dear Mr. Slayden,

To make your life easier, I recommend that you get one or two of your friends to be your liaison, reporting to others. This person should not be your wife, who is already having to answer the same questions many times. Often a person will ask you about your condition, but you are not sure how many details are wanted or understood. Plus, repeating gets difficult. When one of our friends developed cancer, it seemed that no one knew the complete story of his diagnosis. Friends would have to get together to pool information to learn what was going on in his life. A liaison can make this process easier on you, your wife, and your friends. I told my liaison exactly how I felt, what was going on medically, and any setbacks I had. She kept interested people updated. She told friends when I needed extra prayers.

Psalm 46:1 "God is our refuge and strength, a very present help in trouble." (NKJV)

Sincerely,

Lynette

Hi Donna,

Miss Suggestion has returned. These are ideas for around the time of surgery. You have already thought of some of these, but since I do not know which ones, here goes:

(1) Remember to have your arm and body warm whenever they need to stick a vein.

(2) Take colored socks to the hospital to keep your feet warm and clean.

(3) Take your own blanket. Because of the IV drugs, I could not get warm.

(4) Take the notebook so gifts, phone calls, or visits you receive can be recorded.

(5) For when you come home, have ready a basket you'll put all your toiletries in. Include bath items you already use and new items such as first aid tape, gauze, a small pair of scissors, and Vitamin E oil to put on your wound after the bandage comes off. The basket will enable the person who helps you with your shower to easily find everything you need. Since I mentioned the bandage, let me tell you the good news; in the last few years, bandages have really improved. It did not really hurt when the doctor pulled it off.

Our Ladies' Bible class has been praying for you too.

Love,

Lynette

Friends volunteered to take me to chemo. I was very impressed by this type of volunteering. However, when the nurse was inserting the I.V., I did not want to be squeezing on anyone's hand but Morgan's. He made jokes about his hand turning white. During five months, twenty-eight ladies in our congregation made food for us. Some of them made food more than once. If it had not been for them, we would have been malnourished. Many days, chemo makes eating difficult. Morgan would give me small portions and cut my food into extremely tiny bites. I ate five meals a day. Keeping food on my stomach helped me feel better. Day 1, the day I received chemo was when I expected to feel the worst, but usually, I felt worse on Day 3. Other patients have also told me this. Even when I felt nauseous and weak, during the day, I chose to not go to bed. It was better to not isolate myself from my family. It made the days go by a little faster to hear their voices, see their activities, and have their attention. If I had been closed off in the bedroom, days would have become more like the nighttime hours. I spent those days in the recliner surrounded by pillows that made me more comfortable.

While on chemo, eat what appeals to you at that time or what does not make you nauseous. The drugs can sometimes change eating habits. While I did not have cravings as many people do, sweets lost all their appeal. However, I heard of a man who craved animal crackers. On the box he saw the words, "Do not eat if seal is broken." Sure enough, when he opened the box, the giraffe and the elephant were fine, but the seal was chipped, so he could not eat it!

There are precautions a chemo patient must take. Some of the thoughtful people who gave us gifts or food did not know about these precautions. We did not think any less of these givers, since before I had cancer, we did not know these rules either.

While surgery patients can enjoy plants, if a person goes to chemo, plants must be removed. They harbor bacteria that low immunity cannot fight off. Chemo patients must not eat anything raw. Some oncologists let their patients eat raw produce that is peeled, but they still run a risk of bacteria. That means no fresh strawberries, no tossed salads, or other such delights. Chemo patients also often have an exaggerated sense of smell. For the first four days after chemo, the patient should avoid strong fragrances. During those days do not cook chili, Parmesan cheese, garlic, or aromatic concoctions, unless you know that pungent smells do not upset the patient. Often, later in the cycle, scents may not bother the patient. He may even crave strongly flavored foods, especially since some tastebuds can be temporarily destroyed. Chemo also usually affects the patient's digestive system. Foods that are cold or that slide right down are easier to swallow. The drugs can also make a person's lips and nose become dry. I used bendable straws to drink. A patient can use a saline nasal gel or use anti-bacterial Q-tips to administer Vitamin E oil inside nostrils. I preferred extra soft, fragrance-free facial tissues. Some have lotion added. There is also loosely braided dental floss which protects hurting gums. It is called Gentle Care. While on chemo or radiation, the patient's toothbrush should be changed every three weeks. Choose a type with very soft bristles and perhaps a smaller head. You might try a child's version. Some like a battery powered model with a tiny round head, but keep it off painful gums. Morgan bought a humidifier that would be easy to clean and had double tanks to fill with water. He used the little red wagon that our boys had played with as pre-schoolers. Morgan folded a towel into the bottom of the wagon and put the humidifier on top of the towel. During the day we could use the wagon to wheel the moist air machine to the den, but for nighttime we could easily pull it back to the bedroom. If chemo does affect the patient's digestion, I recommend keeping these on hand: Huggies fragrance-free Baby Wipes and either Balmex or Desitin ointment. When my skin became dry, I used Cetaphil moisturizing cream or fragrance-free lotions. During radiation no deodorant which contains aluminum can be used. At that time, some patients use cornstarch in a sugar shaker. Others use deodorants such as Alba Botanic, Tom's of Maine, or Arm and Hammer with Baking Soda.

If it can be arranged, these recommendations will also make the patient's life easier. To assure that the person in treatment gets fewer germs, arrange for him or her to have his own bathroom. Perhaps other family members could use a different bathroom. In addition, clean out the refrigerator to make room for dishes friends will bring. Then have a policy that dishes will be labeled with the date of when each was put in the refrigerator. Otherwise, leftovers will become a mystery. Choose a pharmacy that has a history of personally knowing the customer and his or her needs. This will not be a store which uses a dozen different pharmacists or that prioritizes other things above patient care, understanding, and education. Initiate a real relationship with your pharmacist and tell him of the patient's diagnosis and future needs. The pharmacist can suggest additional items to comfort the person in treatment or discuss possible side-effects of the medications you purchase.

Dear Cayce,

Yes, I also hated my wig, but I was glad that I could afford to buy one. It improved my looks. After wearing it a few hours, even with the liner, it made my head itch. Besides the thin, soft caps I wore at home, the best hat for me while I was out in public was denim with a brim that turned up or down. Onto this hat, I sewed several silk flowers. They were attached to a stem like a vine. I cut the vine to be ten inches long. Then I whip-stitched the vine onto the comfortable hat. Everywhere I wore it, I received many compliments from both men and women. Sometimes I wondered if it "screamed" chemo, and people complimented me because they felt sorry for me. However, as my hair grew back, I kept this hat in the car and used it for a rain hat. While I was buying groceries or walking at the mall, I continued to get compliments from people I did not know. I ordered it from the American Cancer Society catalog. (Visit their website at www.tlccatalog.org or call: 1-800-850-9445.) In addition, when chemo was over but I still had extremely short hair, I bought a couple of inexpensive straw hats. To these I also sewed silk flowers. For another hat I used dried hydrangea blossoms from my backyard. I wove its stem in and out of spaces in the hat. It required no sewing. I guess you have heard that saying regarding perking up your day, "put a flower in your hat." Since right now you cannot be close to real flowers, silk blossoms are a good way to make your day more colorful.

Love,

Lynette

When I am choosing stationery, I always look for colored envelopes, stickers to attach, or I put rubber stamp designs on the edge. The reason is that as soon as the recipient gets the bundle of mail, I want him or her to know that this one is personal and not a bill or junk. I heard of a man who received in the mail an envelope labeled "This is not a bill." He opened it to discover on the inside paper the words, "THIS is the bill!"

1. Will everyone going through the same event have the same experiences?

2. Who invented the oxymoron "miserable comforters?" Why?

3. While we accept the fact that "a word fitly spoken is like apples of gold in settings of silver," are there times when "silence is golden"?

4. In what ways does depending on God go higher and deeper to comfort one than either a perky attitude or assuming you can know the future? (Proverbs 3:5-6)

5. Explain, "God invented details" and the reasons we should tell Him the details of our needs and thanks.

6. Why should adversity be endured in the present and not in the past or the future?

7. List ways to give your prayers your own signature. (Luke 18:1-8; Philippians 4:6-8)

8. For those who are bereaved, depressed, or sick, what type news should a visitor not initiate telling?

9. Where can I go for gift books or tapes that will not become miserable comfort, preach false doctrine, or focus on what could become a burden?

10. Jesus healed many people, but when Paul pleaded for God to take away his "thorn in the flesh," God did not. He told Paul, "My grace is sufficient." What does this tell us about healing? (II Corinthians 12:7-9)

11. Did God leave Paul ill-equipped to flounder on his own?

12. Why is it a good idea to write down medicines taken, the schedule, and side-effects, and good to use a friend as a liaison?

Chapter Ten
Finding Joy Despite Deviating From the Expected

Songs

Tell It To Jesus Alone

His Eye is On the Sparrow

I Traveled Down a Lonely Road

Sing and Be Happy

TodayHeavenly Sunlight

TodayThe Joy of the Lord

I've Got Joy Like a Fountain

There's Not a Friend Like the Lowly Jesus

When All of God's Singers Get Home

You Are the Song That I Sing

My Jesus As Thou Wilt

Sweet Peace

There's Sunshine in My Soul

Sweet Is the Song I'm Singing

There's Within My Heart a Melody

Creator and Sustainer, Please give me the thrill of joy like a fountain.

In Luke 11, Jesus tells the danger of attributing to Satan work done by God. It would also be spiritually dangerous to attribute to God things caused by Satan. The Heavenly Father has gotten a lot of "bad press." Suffering is part of the system of thorns caused by Satan and sin. He also uses it to tempt us, but God tempts no one (James 1:13). Psalm 16 tells us, "You will show me the path of life; in Your presence is fullness of JOY."

Imagine three months you could go nowhere except to the doctor. That was how I spent a winter on chemo which included an epidemic of flu and viruses when germs even closed schools. On trips to the hospital to receive injections to boost my blood, I wore a mask. During my months on chemo I was confined, alone, and did not know what the enemy would do to me. It sounds like being a prisoner of war. However, God created joy out of sorrow. My life's juxtaposition of struggles to joys made the contrast even sweeter and strengthened our faith. My husband grew to appreciate me more, not just because of what I do for him, but because I was his. It caused him to treasure more the vows he made on our wedding day. I was his first priority. Morgan learned skills he had never considered doing. He even rearranged a shelf in one of my cabinets so bowls and lids would fit better. This gave me joy, because his heart was in it. Look for such delights.

Dear Marcia,

Illness can help repriortize a life. I encourage you to keep the New Testament as your standard, not measuring yourself by other people. Even though you have had some difficult days, plan for improvements this will bring to your life through ways you will be more valued, become more in tune with God's plan, and will see more opportunities to serve. I pray that your cancer stays gone, your mind and spirit be soothed, and your relationships with God and loved ones be strengthened.

Psalm 51:12 "Restore to me the joy of Your salvation, and uphold me by Your generous Spirit." (NKJV)

Sincerely,

Lynette

I avoided television news and its disasters, murders, and wars. Where we live cable channels require a satellite dish. I had always said, if one of us became sick, we should get a dish. So, as chemo started, we bought one. While I endured chemo's effects, I watched *The Waltons*, *Andy Griffith*, and *Leave It to Beaver*. Question: What is God's favorite television comedy? Answer: The seven day forecast!

Dear Linda,

God is all-time champion of turning bad times into good. That can include sweet delights, laugh out loud funny moments, as well as the big picture of eternity. Joys you find connected to your ordeal may be different from anything you expected and different from joys I found. It reminds me of the ancient story of the old farmer who knew he would soon die, so he called his sons to his bedside. He said, "Never sell the farm. Somewhere on it is hidden a rich treasure. I do not know the exact spot, but leave no ground unturned in your search." Three times the sons, turned up every inch but found no hidden gold, no silver coins, no jewels, or buried treasure. However, when harvest time came, they had a rich profit far greater than their neighbors, thanks to all their digging. Then they understood that their father's treasure was the wealth of an abundant harvest, and that their hard work had found them the treasure. Spiritually, may you also "dig" and find unexpected treasure!

Romans 15:13 "May the God of hope fill you with all JOY and peace in believing, that you may abound in hope by the power of the Holy Spirit." (NKJV)

Your Sister in Christ,

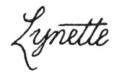

Sisters in Christ collected gifts to make me a Dorcas Basket. I found their treats full of joy. Another patient mentioned that she felt she should send a thank you to each giver of a Dorcas basket gift, but she did not have enough stamina. I encouraged her to send only one thank you to the group.

I received hundreds of cards and saved them in gallon sized, zipper-lock bags. It was extra joyous to receive gifts from ladies who initiated a new friendship. Every thank you card I wrote affirmed God's care for me through His people. I was glad some ladies wrote of their sisters or mothers who went through similar trials and are now "thrivors." Periodically, Alyne Henderson had the Youth Group sign cards. Boone was in the Youth Group, and I was glad they prayed for us. During chemo, several men called me, but Anthony Todd was the only man who sent cards. His wise selections were some of the most tender of any I received. We could tell his cards were not chosen in a hurry.

When it was first announced in Ladies Bible Class that I had cancer and a card was sent around, a friend named Rosemary was so astounded by the news that when she intended to sign her name to the card, she instead put my name. She scribbled this out and wrote in an explanation. I applaud Ladies Bible classes at many congregations where behind the scenes numerous hours of quiet service sometimes go unnoticed. In the spirit of Dorcas, they have soothed, transported, fed, clothed, or encouraged hundreds or thousands.

Dear Laurel Ladies,

I really appreciate the Dorcas Basket of gifts you sent. They were practical, luxurious, for my body, for my mind, and soul. I cherish the thought that went into each selection. Your gestures help me to continue to envision you praying for me, and they are also a wonderful example for Boone and Caleb to see another way of caring in action.

In Christian Love,

Lynette

Dear Fellow Christians in Hartsville,

Thank you for verses you sent which helped you during struggles or telling me how you endured while you were "waiting upon the Lord to renew your strength." Some days I am just longing for chemo's side-effects to pass. Therefore, I still treasure the feelings you pour out to God for me and the compassion you show. You are a blessing to me,

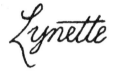

Lynette

I would like to be in a class that investigates the joy found in the teachings of Jesus. I see joyful hope in the often repeated phrase, "Jesus had compassion on the people." This phrase is usually followed by Jesus performing a joyous miracle. There are also probably humorous things Jesus said that we modern Gentiles do not recognize, because we are not familiar with their time, customs, and Greek or Aramaic of the first century. We anticipate Jesus being so serious and spiritual that we readers probably do not look for His joy and humor.

One day while I was in one of my lowest times, I received letters and handmade cards from the Girls' Bible Class I had taught. Lydia and Emily, a couple of the nine-year-olds wrote me this message: "Dear Mrs. Gray, we miss you SO much! We miss you as much as doors would miss not having door-

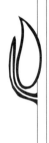

We anticipate Jesus being so serious and spiritual that we readers probably do not look for His joy and humor.

knobs. We miss you as much as books would miss not having pages. We miss you as much as bathrooms would miss not having toilet paper." A laugh burst out of me! I loved their message. It was so sweet, unique, heartfelt, and joyous.

Have you ever been so tired you laughed at weird things—like when you tried to study late at night, but you just got loopy? Our Wellness Community shows a video on laughter's benefits. During chemo, I looked for smiles. Sometimes I needed to laugh at strange things. After three rounds of chemo, my blood counts dropped. I had to begin injections for my immunity. On a Friday, the chemo nurse volunteered to give me Saturday's and Sunday's shots at her family's business and at her home. Her family business turned out to be a dry cleaners. She gave me the injection in my stomach and then a tour of the dry cleaning process. The next day I went to her house. As I sat in a Queen Anne chair with the waist of my slacks pulled below my belly button, because she was slowly injecting the shot, in walked her husband. She began to introduce us, but I would not look his direction, because I did not want to see the shot. I was totally embarrassed, but that also became funny.

These injections enabled my white count to rise 5,000 points in four days. However, after the next chemo, I needed another round of injections. Morgan got a cold with a terrible cough but insisted on driving me to get the shots, so I wore a mask. When we arrived at the almost empty waiting room, I sat far away and removed my mask. Morgan kept motioning to me. Finally, he whispered, "You have make-up streaks beside your mouth. I replied, "I don't have on any make-up! It's the lines from wearing the mask." The next day, I drove us to the hospital without the mask and had Morgan sit in the very back of the minivan, hoping his germs would not reach me. We were a sorry sight, as sick people taking care of one another in weird ways. We laughed. More laughs came when during chemo, I was summoned to jury duty. Joyfully, I was excused.

Dear Kay,

My sister Twyla tells me that your mouth has been hurting. Here is a recipe for a nutritious salad that is good when your mouth is tender. Your husband can even make it.

Another thing that helps a sore mouth or throat is a pre-scription of Magic Mouthwash. It helps to heal and numb. It is thick, but I would gargle it to keep it on my problem area as long as possible. As I gargled, my reflexes made me cough, spraying it all over the bathroom mirror. Therefore, hold a wash cloth in front of your mouth. Now, I can smile when I think of that.

Psalm 126:3 and 5 "The Lord has done great things for us, and we are glad. Those who sow in tears shall reap in joy." (NKJV)

I pray that you are seeing God's daily blessings. However, I have to pray often that I will have my eyes and heart open to see them, touch them, taste them, and hear them, but NOT smell them. (HA!) That is a little chemo humor. It is hard to find.

Your Sister, *Lynette*

LYNETTE'S FROZEN FRUIT SALAD

1 can cherry pie filling (OR try peach or blueberry)

20 oz. can crushed pineapple (include juice)

1 can sweetened condensed milk

1/4 cup lemon juice

1 can Mandarin oranges (any size; NO juice)

Mix all ingredients. Line muffin tins with paper liners. Pour. When frozen, store in air tight container. Label and get out only as many as need-ed. Thaw 10 minutes before serving.

Dear Emma Lou,

If you need a chuckle, let me set the stage. My son Boone weighs 135 pounds and is six feet and two inches tall. Yes, he is a "string bean," but he is a speedy runner. This morning I had writ-ten to you and Leah and Nita, two other ladies who are also fight-ing cancer. Boone was doing homework when he said, "Mom, the mail just came." I said, "Oh, no! Leslie's early; I didn't get those let-ters to the box." Boone asked if I wanted him to chase her as she went away from our end of the road. I said I doubted he could run that fast. Our driveway is long.

Well, Boone still had on his pajamas—a Kermit the Frog T-shirt and red Long-Johns. As he ran out of the house in a flash, he said the only shoes he could get into quickly were his elf shoes. In December, Boone had been a Santa elf. His footwear were size 11 slip-on canvas shoes to which I had sewn padded curled-up toes and completely overlaid in shiny red duct tape. Then I attached sparkly green tassels. Boone was half way to the road when the mail lady pulled out of the neighbor's driveway. Boone sped up. She put mail in a box that was farther away. Boone increased his strides as she drove to another mailbox and one more distant still. Boone really poured on the speed as Leslie started up a long hill. He ran like a gazelle, looked like a clown, and waved the three letters. He was even gaining on her as she ascended the incline. Then she stopped and gave a "beep, beep" on the horn. She was laughing. She told Boone she thought he was just a runner until she saw he was gaining on her car and that he was waving mail. She laughed more. Boone tried to speak, but, he was very out of breath. He explained his weird outfit. Leslie replied that she thought he had on running tights. However, Boone never did comment on his elf shoes that she had now spotted. I bet this comic scene gave Leslie Choy's family several things to discuss at dinner.

Feel special. I am not the only one who has an investment in letters I send you. Sometimes Boone has put his skills to work also. Value humor to help you smile during the unpleasant, cope with the unexpected, tolerate the unbearable, and overlook the embarrassing.

Lovingly,

Lynette

Sometimes joys come from being able to negotiate with my doctor. I can write about making deals with a doctor because I have doctors whom I can trust to be well educated, medically up-to-date, willing to explain things to me, and not having a philosophy that cancer is only localized. However, contrary to the attitudes of a few doctors in my distant past, I am glad to say my physicians give me individual care that is tailor-made for my uniquenesses. They not only discuss treatment alternatives, they are willing to think on their feet, and even change their minds. Some people who know they need surgery or treatments actually interview other patients and their physicians. Choose a doctor who suits your specific needs. They are the doctors, and I am not. Once I had chosen a physician, I never tried to negotiate decisions that only the doctor should decide, but when it came to slight changes in scheduling, location, or comfort, I could play "Let's Make a Deal" with my oncologist.

Dear Ken,

I am not writing to Susan today. I do not want her to worry. However, if this situation arises, you will be able to comfort her. I did not know it was a real probability, until it happened to me.

I had heard that some people on chemo take growth factor, but I thought it was for people who have bone marrow transplants or for really old ladies. While it is true that growth factor is for these, it is used on younger people too. One weekly injection is to stimulate bone marrow to make red blood cells, which usually take 120 days to be manufactured. Another shot is to stimulate bone marrow to make white cells which usually take only a week to be made. It is given daily for four to ten days. Red cells carry oxygen and contribute to stamina. White cells boost immunity.

The nurse assumed I would give myself these shots in the stomach. I gently, emphatically said no. Then she assumed Morgan would give them. She had the video ready to teach him how. I said, "We need to talk." She knelt down beside me. I told her that Morgan has absolutely no medical experience. I did not want to blame him for pain and wonder if he did something wrong. We found out that the hospital could give the shots. That is what we did for ten days. Their usual schedule is to begin the blood boosting shots on the same day as a chemo treatment. I reasoned that because my white count was not dropping immediately after chemo, and because I had always felt worse on Day 3, could I please delay beginning the next cycle of daily blood-booster shots until Day 4 after chemo. That worked out much better. There truly is an UP side. When chemo was over, I am certain that I bounced back faster because of the blood booster injections.

Sincerely,

Lynette

Recently I learned of a possible option to taking bone marrow booster shots. Ask your oncologist to investigate work by Drs. Georges Maestroni, Augusto Pedrazzini, David Blask, and Russel Reiter on melatonin.

As a young adult how did you envision your future? Cancer showed me I could play a role I never dreamed I was capable of. Even though I became a person who limped along in the theatrical production of life, I was grateful to still be a player. Roles have changed in the past and can change again in the future. One trait most centenarians posses is the ability to adapt to new situations. God can even empower a person who thought she could not adapt. Ask Him to help you be malleable and have Christ's attitudes also become yours.

Hebrews 12:12-13 "So take a new grip with your tired hands, stand firm on your shaky legs, and mark out a straight, smooth path for your feet so that those who follow you, though weak and lame, will not fall and hurt themselves, but become strong." (The Living Bible)

While on chemo, I knew I was doing everything possible to battle cancer. My only job was to endure. Once treatments were over, I did not know whether all enemy cells were dead. The amount of cards dwindled, so I guessed prayers had dwindled also. Then I was put on a drug to reduce the chances that cancer would return. Being again atypical, after three weeks, it crippled me and affected my mind and speech. I was taken off of it. Most of the side-effects left immediately. However, my bone pain lingered. Eventually, I had to try another drug to thwart cancer's return. I had to be taken off of it also. In the midst of all this, I was able to begin going back to worship services on Sunday nights. Since people were seeing me out, they assumed a certain schedule for me. One evening a man asked if I felt better than I had the week before. I told him that I did not. (I felt worse, because I had just begun the new drug, but I did not say that.) He announced I was not feeling better. I was embarrassed. Chemo's end will not mean the person is instantly back to her pre-cancer self. Whether your struggle is with extended illness, grief, or relationships, do not insist upon a certain schedule.

Dear Bonnie,

No matter how much I have warned myself to be braced for bad news, it still takes me off-guard. Keep up hope even if news is not as good as you wished. Oncologists can predict what happens to a group in similar circumstances to yours, but they have no crystal ball to know what will happen to one individual. An oncologist may be an authority on the types of treatments he gives but is not an expert on every treatment. Keep praying that God puts you in the hands of the right people and the correct information. During chemo your mind and body may not be equipped to investigate cancer yourself. Perhaps a relative would be willing to invest the time it would take to research adjuvant therapies (something that enhances the results of another treatment). Usually adjuvant treatments cannot begin until chemo is over. Be sure books, articles, or Internet information that you read are current and well-balanced. For example, I read books and articles from physicians, cancer patients, American authors, Europeans, conservative writers, and the avant guard of medicine, congressional hearings, the American Cancer Society, and the National Cancer Institute. Reading only one type source can skew your view.

For adjuvant therapy, I was to take a drug that purportedly would reduce the chances of cancer returning. Keep in mind I have always been extraordinarily sensitive to drugs. After learning the benefits and risks of the specific pharmaceutical I was prescribed, I prayed, "God, please show me abundantly clearly whether I should take it or not. If I would be harmed by it, or if I do not need it, show me not to take it." Most definitely, my oncologist and I were shown in many ways that I could not take the drug. When my research became more intense, I was delighted to discover natural lifestyle changes a person can make to help diminish her chances of cancer. In place of the pharmaceuticals I could not take, several foods, supplements, exercise, and avoidances can accomplish good things and also enhance general health.

Even if you have a troubling diagnosis, your fate is not sealed! Acknowledge the diagnosis, but do not accept a certain prognosis as your verdict. We humans tend to acknowledge God but focus on the problems. In contrast, recognize your enemies, but *focus* on the love and power of God and any creative solutions He can provide a seeker.

Ephesians 3:20-21 "Now to Him who is able to do immeasurably more than all we ask or imagine, according to His power that is at work within us, to Him be glory in the church and in Christ Jesus throughout all generations, for ever and ever! Amen" (NIV)

Sincerely,

Lynette

Not every person who suffers through illness will be healed during this lifetime. However, each child of God in relationship with Him will be given a new body that never needs healing. No one will enter heaven limping, wheezing, or pushing an I.V.! Truly acknowledging and accepting the cross and empty tomb of Jesus Christ does not let a person deny the love and power of God.

Dear Willadean,

These are my experiences that your letter brought back to mind. When I expected to feel bad, for example right after a chemo treatment, I was prepared for it physically and emotionally. People who inquired seemed to also expect this schedule. In contrast, when I had times I did not expect to feel as bad as I did, my unpreparedness "threw me for a loop."

While in chemo, do not measure yourself by past productivity. Sometimes we almost canonize quotes like: "Cleanliness is next to Godliness." God did not say that. We should not try to be dirty, but we emphasize the physical too much. During this time, relinquish old expectations. Even though you may not be able to mop or take care of others right now, you can be productive; you are being trained on how to see with new perspective and focus. Your spiritual eyes can open wider and become more astute. Don't settle for the world's priorities. This is your time as a sheep of the Good Shepherd to ruminate. Therefore, pray, sing, ask God questions, listen for His answers....All that is a different and more timely type productivity. Praying for you daily,

Lynette

Dear Carole,

The message was relayed to me that you have had bronchitis and became discouraged. I know that feeling very well. I am glad that you're better.

Difficult times cause some people to run to God and other people to run from Him. I believe that part of the reason for this is the perspective of one's heart. For example, to people who want to believe in evolution, looking at the similarities between a fish and a bird causes them to attribute the similarities to evolution. Conversely, people who do not believe in evolution, looking at the similarities among animals, causes them to attribute the similarities to the fact that there is one Creator. The different response is not because of the power of the information they are shown, but a different perspective of the heart. Either view requires faith.

As an artist, this is how I see the phrase "difference in perspective." Look around the room where you are sitting and then stand up and go several feet to the side. I remember having dusted a room and then climbing up on a stool and seeing the tops of tall furniture and thinking how inadequate my dusting had been. When my perspective changed, I saw many things I had not seen earlier. Suffering can also change our perspective. Even so, experience does not make people wiser; it is what a person does with the experience that makes her wiser.

In difficult times some individuals seek God, while others deny His power, spurn His love, and blame Him for what we do not understand. In Exodus 14, as the Israelites left Egypt they were guided by God's presence in a cloud by day and a pillar of fire at night. This pillar of fire stood between the Israelites and Egyptians who pursued them. To God's people it was a guiding light, but to their enemies it was blackness which blocked their view. The New Testament has a similar idea. When Jesus is asked why He teaches in parables, He says that for some people parables will make His teachings more understandable, but parables will confuse others. (Matthew 13:11-13) I perpetually ask God to give your heart and mine the proper perspective and to sharpen our spiritual focus. He is the divine ophthalmologist.

Yours Truly,

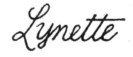

Dear Wanda,

While in the midst of treatments, I introduced myself to several television shows I had never seen. One such program was on HGTV and revolved around decorating and the focus of a room with challenges. Cameras would go to a home that had misused space. Then two interior designers would completely empty the room and rearrange the belongings. This would usually give the room a different focus, feeling, and flow. Sometimes they would even cart in an item from the garage, but they were not allowed to purchase new items. The improvements were phenomenal. This makes me think of a God-guided life. While you struggle, remember that *real* hope is not because of a certain medical fact or a particular circumstance. Real hope is in God, and He can arrange my life and yours so much better than we can. He can take the same circumstances, my same struggles, your same talents or fears and bring phenomenal improvements. Besides the fact that the room (my life) will have new focus, and now function, flow, and feel better, God can even incorporate items from the "garage"—stuff I had forgotten about, had under-used, or did not know I had.

God is the interior designer who arranges and decorates. He can give you new focus and enhance your functions. You or I can resist Him and keep control ourselves. Or, we can see the great hope in giving God complete control. May God help you see the hope and bless your "focus," "arranging," and "decorating" challenges.

Yours Truly,

Lynette

Dear Fred,

Psalm 126:5 "They that sow in tears, shall reap in joy."

Author Craig Larson uses events in the life of speed skater, Dan Jansen to exemplify perseverance. Dan first competed at the Olympics in 1984 when he skated the 500 meter and the 1,000 meter races. At age eighteen, he finished fourth in the 500 meters.

He missed the bronze medal by just sixteen one-hundredths of a second.

Four years later, while Dan was waiting to skate Calgary's Olympic 500 meter race, his brother called saying their sister Jane was dying of leukemia, but she asked Dan to skate for her. Just prior to the race, Dan received word that Jane had died. When race time came, he fell. In the 1,000 meter race four days later, he fell again. He had never fallen in a race.

Since the 500 meter race was his specialty, it was anticipated that Dan would win it at the 1992 Olympics. However, he finished fourth in that race and performed pitifully in the 1,000.

Years later, at what was expected to be his last chance to win any Olympic race, Dan's left foot lost its balance in the final turn and he touched the ice with his hand. It slowed him down to eighth place and devastated him.

Dan knew that there was only one race left between him and retirement. Near the end of the race, fans gasped when Dan slipped and caught his fall by touching his hand to the ice. After Dan crossed the finish line, he looked up to a scoreboard that proclaimed " World Record" beside his name.

It didn't happen the way he expected, when he anticipated, or through the event that was predicted, but Dan Jansen had finally won the highest medal. Through years of training and practice, eight Olympic races, and a decade of losing, Dan had chased that gold medal. Then someone put a simple home made sign in the snow on the side of the main road from Lillehammer. It said, "Dan." It said so much more.

Fred, to me the comfort of this story is that God knows your name and mine. He knows the obstacles you have overcome, the striving you have done, the disappointments you have suffered, the scars you have acquired, the example you have been. He has washed you whiter than snow and written your name in the Lamb's Book of Life.

Your Sister,

Lynette

In order to find something extra to anticipate, some patients plan a trip or a special delight for several weeks later. The importance of this novel pleasure may be in the dreaming as much as in the attainment. Other times, it is a loved one who secretly plans a particularly personal gift or event to celebrate the end of treatments and to demonstrate love. Envision this pleasure all you want to during those bad times, but do not schedule its fruition before your body is recovered enough to truly enjoy the thrill.

Dear Cayce,

Most chemo patients are very anxious to get back to their former ways of life. Yes, like them I longed to be able to once again eat certain prohibited foods, go out in crowds, and regain stamina, but I never longed to get back to my former ways of life exactly as they had been. The discerning reflections that came with cancer's shocking announcement, my floundering, pondering, and praying caused me to see improvements my former life needed.

A life-threatening disease has lessons to teach that cannot be read in a book or heard in a sermon. It has prayers to utter that are not spoken in public worship nor around most dinner tables. It has songs to sing that are on no sheet music or CD. Extended illness can bring alterations not only to a spiritual life, but also other areas. However, these lessons, prayers, songs, and alterations are not forced upon one nor guaranteed. Improvements that come to you as a result of your illness are because you decided to grow and not resist. They come from truly desiring to be malleable clay in God's hands. The words human and humble both come from the same Latin root word which means earth; we are dust. Psalm 100:3 "Know that the Lord, He is God; it is He who has made us, and not we ourselves." (NKJV) We function best when we connect with the Creator and grow in the fullness of His divinely planned ultimates.

If you have ever watched Carol Duvall on HGTV, you know that her guests often teach how to make items with polymer clay. To prevent cracks and explosions in the heating process, they advise that you never begin until you have conditioned the clay at least thirty times. Off screen, they have mashed, smashed, rolled, and folded. Then the clay has been perpetually refolded and run through a pasta machine until all bubbles and imperfections are worked out. It is the job of the clay to "go with the flow," and in this case to also go with the fold.

Isaiah 29:16 "Can the pot say to the Potter, 'He knows nothing?' "

Isaiah 45:9 "Does the clay say to the Potter, 'What are You making?' "

Be reassured that the Potter will never bully you, tempt you, or forsake you. He conditions clay to make it supple, adaptable, useful, beautiful, and enduring. I certainly want those qualities, so I must leave the process in the Potter's hands. He totally knows how to put into us and bring out of us the best we can be.

Your friend,

Lynette

Dear John,

Any season is a good time to be getting over sickness or treatments, but spring is extra great. As the plants come back to life, so can you. However, if some days you do too much and do not fit the schedule you had hoped for, concentrate on your new hope, not on a delay. God's "manna" is not to encourage one to ask what He will do for the next day or the next week. It is like the phrase in the Lord's Prayer where Jesus prays for daily bread. I do not believe that He was talking only about bread. He could have meant any daily sustenance, even spiritual bread.

As you prepare for your new adventure to resume your regular life, consider when Jesus healed the lame man and said, "Rise, take up your bed and walk." John, you are about the "walk," but don't forget to "take up your bed." The bed is a reminder of, how it is to be ill, be reminded of sickness' memories that can improve the joy of the "walk," and be reminded of new blessings, and helping others. Ponder all the ways you will "take up your bed." Then be cheered that everyone is so thrilled to know you are about ready to be back with us in your "walk."

In Christian Love,

1. How can God give His people joy even in suffering? (John 16:31-32; Romans 15:4-6 & 13; Galatians 5:22-23; Philippians 1:21)

2. List objects that could be put into a Dorcas basket.

3. What does a smile or a laugh do for a hurting or sick person? (Proverbs 17:22)

4. Can you name a joyous or funny event that happened to you in the midst of calamity?

5. When we get a preconceived notion of exactly how God should solve our troubles, how do we limit God? (Ephesians 3:20)

6. Tell how one's perspective makes all the difference while seeing the cloud of God's presence at the Red Sea or hearing parables which enlightened some and confused others. (Exodus 14:19-20; Matthew 13:10-11; II Corinthians 4:3-4)

7. As Providence, how does God arrange, focus, and decorate our lives? (Most of our children have never heard God called Providence.)

8. In what ways can a car wreck, prolonged illness, or a near death experience actually improve a person?

9. What does the potter do to the clay to make it malleable? Toward what purpose?

10. What are the rights of the clay? (Isaiah 29:16; 45:9)

11. What are God's purposes for us, the clay?

12. Explore the full meaning of, "Rise, take up your bed and walk." (John 5:7-8)

Chapter Eleven
Looking Back and Seeing God's Fingerprints

Songs

He Leadeth Me

I Know Who Holds the Future

Blest Be the Tie That Binds

Jesus Hold My Hand

Have You Seen Jesus My Lord

Our Heavenly Father Understands

Because He Lives

Let the Beauty of Jesus Be Seen in Me

In Heavenly Love Abiding

He Keeps Me Singing

God Who Stretched the Spangled

Beyong This Land of Parting

My God and I

No Tears in Heaven

Living By Faith

Great God of heaven, Endow my eyes and heart to look back and see ways You took care of me even beyond what I realized at the time, and let this give me hope.

We have all read the mystery novels or seen television police shows. When and why do detectives look for fingerprints? They look for fingerprints after the event has happened to decide who is responsible. Similarly, it is often difficult to see God's fingerprints until later. It may be a few hours later or many years later. God's fingerprints become evident after He turns a bad situation into good. Look at the book of Job where Satan caused the suffering, but God slowly turned it into good. Concerning my cancer, I can see many instances of God exposing me to the right information or guiding my feet, eyes, ears, and heart.

Dear Diane,

It is very likely that sometime during your struggles with cancer, you have asked yourself why this happened and what does it mean. Solomon, the wisest king who ever lived spent decades researching the meaning of life and the reasons behind why a certain event happens. In Ecclesiastes we see his almost scientific journal of what he tried and observed. Solomon questions life's unfairness. His investigations are neither myopic nor short-lived.

I Kings 4:28-34: "God gave Solomon wisdom and very great insight, and a breath of understanding as measureless as the sand on the seashore....He was wiser than any other man....He spoke thousands of proverbs and his songs numbered a thousand and five. He described plant life, from the cedar of Lebanon to the hyssop that grows out of walls. He also taught about animals and birds, reptiles and fish. Men of all nations came to listen to Solomon's wisdom, sent by all the kings of the world, who had heard of his wisdom." (NIV)

In his God-given wisdom, Solomon rejects trite, easy answers or conventional replies to life's problems. While other so-called wise men might be sure that they know why God lets certain things happen, Solomon understands that their confidence does not mean they are correct. Over dozens of years, spending probably millions of dollars, and investigating both physical and mental labor, this is what Solomon finds: pleasures, work, riches, and even education are meaningless in the grand scheme of things. We are not in control, and many things that happen in this world are frustrating. Ecclesiastes 3:11 "God has put eternity in the heart of men, yet they cannot fathom what God has done." (NIV)

Our duty is not to insist we can decipher what only God can discern, but to fit into God's purposes and accept life as a gift. This will include fun events and miserable situations. Even if we grow to feel useless, remember—this life is not all there is. In all his wisdom, Solomon does not claim to understand why evil people sometimes prosper or why good people suffer. Solomon preaches that we should enjoy life, not because it always follows our limited view of fairness, but because life is short, a gift from God, and to the glory of the Creator. If our request is not answered as we wanted, then it must be that God has something better in mind for us. Remember, He is working everything *together* for our good.

Ecclesiastes 12:13-14 "Fear God and keep His commandments, for this is the whole duty of man. For God will bring every deed into judgement, including every hidden thing, whether good or evil." (NIV) Thus there are no throw-away moments. Life is still a precious gift. The highest wisdom is to face the facts that we are each His creation and a player on God's stage. The Lord is Sovereign, Creator, Providence, and Good.

Regardless of why cancer came, God can use it to accomplish something wonderful that currently seems to have no connection to your struggles. Look for God's fingerprints. He loves you dearly. Envision yourself "Safe in the Arms of Jesus." May your heart smile.

Your sister in Christ and your sister in struggles,

Lynette

Dear Donna,

Your e-mail shocked me. In gigantic letters above each of our lives should be the words, "On this side of eternity we'll never understand why what happens does happen!" You and I are prevention and solution people. We investigate, ponder, and take actions to prevent calamity. If that doesn't work, we do the same procedure to find remedies. Maybe we have been too prone to believe a certain thing happened to a person BECAUSE of what she did or didn't do. Sometimes things happen IN SPITE of all you or I do. One lesson is: we cannot anticipate all the possibilities. However, that statement should not be given only negative connotations. We cannot anticipate all the wonderfully fabulous things God causes to happen, many of which we did not even know He had arranged: calamities from which He saved us, pains He took away, friends He sent, information He made available, doctors He enabled, insights He gave, car wrecks that missed us, Bible verses He brought to our attention, songs He put in our hearts, and faith He helped us grow. I believe that is the true soothing and comfort of Matthew 10:30 which says that God knows the number of hairs on your head. It is not really about hairs. It is saying that God knows your exact composition. He made you unique and knows all the sciences of Donna's body. He INVENTED Science. Smile. God's verse about hair pertains to you even now with no hair.

Love,

Lynette

Remember, my friend Martha advised that we pray for God to put the right people in our lives. When I had gone for mammograms in the 1990s, I had gone to a certain mammography center. I had never seen a doctor there, just technicians. However, October 6, 2000, after finding the lump the night before, I called this place for a mammogram and was told they could not see me for two weeks. My heart fell as I looked up unknown places in the Yellow Pages, but within ten minutes, the center with my records called back saying they had a cancellation and could see me the next day! I told no one, went alone, had a mammogram and an ultrasound. As the RN prepared me for the biopsy, she told me they also have a surgeon who does cancer surgery. She said his name was Dr. Webber, and he is so kind and informative with his patients that their visits often take longer than the staff anticipates. Well, that sounded like my kind of person, but I was skeptical of a place that had this cancer treatment organized into a neat business package.

Then the radiologist performed the biopsy and told me it was definitely cancer. I wiped my tears, caught my breath, and drove myself home. I made an appointment for my husband and me to have a conference with my gynecologist, Dr. Pierce. Even though cancer is not his field, we trusted him to take time with us and to advise us in ways that we could not anticipate. Knoxville has several oncology surgeons, but I had only vaguely heard of two. I asked my gynecologist about these two. He said patients of his had used both of these surgeons. Even though he would make no recommendation of a certain surgeon to choose, he advised us to consider the ramifications of what hospital each one uses. He also advised that I learn to very much "stay in the day." Then he recommended that I also be tested for cancer that could have traveled to other specific places in my body.

Twenty-two years ago, Morgan and I had been in a home Bible study group with several couples including George and Peggy. Eighteen years ago Peggy had breast cancer. Six months before my cancer was discovered Peggy's husband George had died. As soon as I told our congregation I had cancer, Peggy called to console me and pray with me. It was the first time I had ever been involved in a telephone prayer. I told her my quandary of not knowing which surgeon to choose. She said that since her son is a physician at the same hospital as Dr. Webber, whom I was considering, she would page her son and ask his opinion. She did. Peggy told me that her son said he highly recommended Dr. Webber. They had been in the operating room together, and he admired Dr. Webber's work. I decided to choose Dr. Webber as my surgeon, but that was only the beginning of seeing the fingerprints of God as He directed me and put the right people in my life.

The first day I met Dr. Webber, he walked into the room, smiled, and said, "I'm very sorry to meet you!" He explained that he wished we could have met under better circumstances, even maybe at a party. He was reassuring. He had his nurse take a photo of me to attach to my patient file, so whenever I might call that office, the nurse or doctor would know the exact person with whom they were speaking. They would be counseling or prescribing for my specific needs, not for a generic being. Dr. Webber also took us into a conference room where he explained the procedures, jargon, and expectations. He drew on a marker board, answered our questions, and showed a video. He gave me choices between two types of surgery and what day to schedule it. Dr. Webber also kindly assured me that if I needed him during the middle of the night, to call.

I vaguely remember Dr. Webber telling me that at that time, he was the only surgeon in our city who did a new diagnostic procedure to tell him whether lymph nodes should be removed. He inserts a dye into sentinel nodes. I thought no more about this for ten months. That is when my brother's wife was diagnosed with breast cancer. She called and told me she was thrilled to have found the only surgeon in her much larger city who is on the cutting-edge and does a new test on lymph nodes using sentinel node dye! That is when my appreciation for Dr. Webber stepped up another notch. That is when my appreciation for God's fingerprints stepped up another notch. Remember, I kept praying that He would put the right people in my life.

A few days after surgery, while my husband and I sat in Dr. Webber's waiting room, an older lady came up to Morgan and called his name. This woman's name is Marie. She had brought a friend to the doctor. When Morgan was in graduate school, Marie had been the secretary of his major professor. Marie said many years earlier, Dr. Webber had performed abdominal surgery on her husband. Dr. Webber then prescribed that Marie's husband rock daily in a rocking chair. Marie said at the time this was unheard of, but Dr. Webber told them that when a person has been under anesthesia, his organs can wake up on different schedules; rocking would help them all wake up. Marie said now, many renowned hospitals have their surgery patients rock.

A lady from Reach to Recovery came to my house to give me some literature and items from the American Cancer Society. She had never seen anyone as agile as I was so soon after a mastectomy and lymph node removal. She also had never seen a patient wear the binder that Dr. Webber has his patients wear. It is like a tight tube-top with Velcro up the front. He says it is to hold the surgery back against the chest wall. It also helped me feel protected against injury. I think it helped speed my recovery. Again, God left His fingerprints.

Dr. Webber told me to make an appointment at a certain hospital supply store to be fitted for a prosthesis. He warned that experiences at another such store across town could be negative. At the store the doctor recommended, the lady who fitted me said that after doing this many years, she knew I was far ahead of schedule in speed of recovery. She said Dr. Webber's patients nearly always seem to bounce back sooner. She told me that before each surgery he prays for himself and for that lady. God kept leaving fingerprints.

Unlike at some clinics or hospitals, my radiologist, surgeon, and oncologist have a conference about each patient's further care. It reassured me to know that I did not have just one person making decisions for me. We had a conference with the oncologist, Dr. Brig, concerning my chemo. In the meantime, I found out that as a teenager Dr. Brig had Ewing's Sarcoma himself. This contributed to his being sympathetic. I later saw Dr. Brig do several things that many doctors refuse to do. I witnessed him treat me as an individual whose systems often do not conform to what books predict will be the "normal" reaction to certain drugs. Once, I enjoyed seeing him get very quiet after listening to what I said, and then tell me that he needed to think about what I had said. He pondered and decided that if I did what he had first advised, my fragile veins might have to go through an extra blood test, so he adapted my schedule for me to skip one extra blood test that was not necessary. That is a big deal to over-used veins. There are those fingerprints of God.

After going into each examining room, Dr. Brig goes out to a tape recorder and speaks into it, to summarize his diagnosis and record what he prescribed. On one occasion, the room next to mine was occupied by an attractive lady of about seventy-five, who had cancer a few years earlier. When Dr. Brig went to his tape recorder, I heard him include in his assessment of her the fact that her husband had recently died. That is all that I heard, but I was very impressed that he was treating the whole person, not just looking at her as having cancer or not having cancer. It told me that he knew the loss of her husband had the possibility of causing a change of outlook in her life, thus affecting her fight against cancer.

At each visit to Dr. Brig, I took questions. He patiently answered. I would type out when I took any medicine and my reaction to each prescription. He would read these facts and comment, explain, or make suggestions. I asked my husband once if he thought that any of Dr. Brig's other patients asked questions like mine. Morgan said, "Absolutely not; nobody asks questions like you!"

Each of these incidences reaffirmed to me that God had put the right people into my life and had opened my eyes of faith to see the requests answered. I have often told God, "Please, make Your answer very obvious; I'm not too bright about recognizing whether it was from you." Thank you God for Your fingerprints!

Dear Nita,

I often pray that my words will speak to your specific needs and timetable. May today's tidings bring you hope, love, and peace. Two years ago, between Thanksgiving and Christmas, I was to begin chemo. I feared the unknown, the drug reactions, needles, vein problems, difficulties with blood, the lack of estrogen, my inabilities to do certain things, how my family might handle chemo, the pain, what to tell people, and being so out of control. Up until that time, my life was usually so happy that I always have had plans I wanted to see fulfilled or children I wanted to see succeed in their activities. I have wanted God to delay His coming back so we could have more earthly pleasures or so that I could get myself more ready for His coming. However, anticipating chemo, I was so afraid, I asked God that if He were going to end the world any time soon, could he please do it BEFORE I started chemo. Then I knew that I had to get myself ready. Before I could begin the action of getting ready for the end of time, I needed to ponder exactly what I needed to do to get ready. I prayed that I would know the answers to my needs. Using scripture, I saw I needed to study grace more, truly comprehend it better, and concentrate on the specifics of how the loving God of the Bible would handle a repeat sinner like me.

To visualize the relationship, I made up analogies of what an attentive and adoring parent would do in certain situations. I applied them to my life with God. I saw that Satan has tried to use my own guilt to distance me from God, and Satan has used my shyness to convince me to sometimes not speak up for Christ. Next, God showed me that if I were going to get ready for death, I needed to also get ready to live! After all, getting ready for death is what best equips one to really live! This required that I begin living with a passion for Jesus I should have had all along. Satan knows that my guilt and my shyness can be combined to rob me of Godly enthusiasm. Then I looked at those precious Old Testament characters—people who loved God, struggled to follow Him, and changed the history of a nation or even the world. Yet, in their lives I see selfish, manipulative, stupid, or fearful actions. I can identify with those!

Jacob, for example was a "mama's boy" who hung around the tent, as a conniving sneak who took advantage of his desperate brother on one occasion, cheated him on another, and tricked their old blind father. After Jacob fled for his life, he laid down at Bethel to sleep. There he saw angels ascending and descending a ladder or ramp to heaven. What was Jacob motivated to do with this miraculous visitation and knowledge? Think of the humble and respectful reactions he could have had. Instead, Jacob decided to haggle with God. Of course, we do not know how much Jacob knew about God and His nature, but the deal seems rather naive, arrogant, and regulating. Jacob said that if God would keep him safe on his journey to Haran and back, give Him food to eat, new clothes to wear, and return him in good condition to Isaac's house, THEN Jacob would make the Lord his God!

How did this pampered con man become a hard working responsible person who feared God and leaned on Him without making a deal? Possibly it was Jacob's gradual maturity and his love for Rachel. The first time Jacob saw Rachel, he even cried. His love for her was not just being in love with love, nor merely passion. He did not love her only for what they had in common or what they did not. Jacob was totally "head over heels" in love with Rachel in every way, so much that when his agreed upon seven years of working for her ended, "it seemed as only a few days." Jacob could have received a larger dowry to marry Laban's first-born daughter Leah, but in spite of riches, he wanted Rachel. Even when Jacob was completely bamboozled by the trio of Laban, Leah, and Rachel, he still wanted Rachel. His love and devotion to Rachel was evident to all. Even when after years of marriage and Rachel could bear him no children, he still loved her the most. Later, when God "opened her womb," her sons were extra special to Jacob also.

Years ago, I heard Ken Chaffin ask the question, "Is God your Rachel or your Leah?" Chaffin characterized Jacob's love for Leah as duty, doing what he knew he should, keeping his obligations, providing for her, but nothing devoted. In contrast, Jacob's love for Rachel was deep, burning, impassioned, embellished, all-involving, invigorating, second-to-none, and life-long. Is God my Rachel or my Leah? Yes, I had done the right things, followed the rules, and been dutiful, but I had not known the enthusiasm for God that Jacob felt for Rachel. It took cancer to humble me, make me ponder, insist that I take the time to make things right, study grace, and become EAGER for God. Hymns and gospel songs have helped me too.

Romans 12:1-2, 11-12: "Therefore, I urge you, brothers, in view of God's mercy, to offer your bodies as living sacrifices, holy and pleasing to God— this is your spiritual act of worship. Do not conform any longer to the pattern of this world, but be transformed by the renewing of your mind. Then you will be able to test and approve what God's will is— His good, pleasing and perfect will....Never be lacking in zeal, but keep your spiritual fervor, serving the Lord. Be joyful in hope, patient in affliction, faithful in prayer." (NIV)

Compassionately,

Lynette

One night years later, as Jacob took his wives and children to meet his brother Esau, Jacob wrestled with God. The Almighty changed Jacob's name to Israel which means "struggles with God." Do not consider yourself unique when you struggle with God or your perceptions of Him. Talk to Him more, and let Him design and deliver answers to your questions.

Dear Kay,

Last week, my son Boone was at Hillbrook Christian Camp. He heard one of the counselors pray for Kay Hughes. So, afterwards, Boone went up to him and said, "I know Kay Hughes!"

Because Boone had heard me mention you so very often, he felt as if he knew you. It is all the more remarkable when you know how thoroughly awful Boone is at remembering names. I hope it makes you feel loved and makes you know that you are on God's mind and in His care because of Christians praying for you!

Psalm 86:15, 17: "You, O Lord, are a compassionate and gracious God, slow to anger, abounding in love and faithfulness. You, O Lord have helped me and comforted me." (NIV)

I Corinthians 2:9: "No eye has seen, no ear has heard, no mind has conceived what God has prepared for those who love Him." (NIV)

In Christian Love,

Lynette

Dear Marlyn,

Last fall, as I read Randy Becton's book *Everyday Strength*, he recommended writings by J.B. Phillips on discouragement. Our county library occasionally has old books for sale. They are the dregs, like out-dated computer books or how to speak ancient Choctaw. After reading Randy's book, the next time I went to the library, in with fifty used books that were rejects, sat *365 Meditations* by Phillips. It was twenty-five cents and had the section Randy recommended. I bought it. A dozen pages I have marked to go back and reread later. My point is: I was not looking for this book. It was unexpected, but I am very glad I found it. Maybe God put it in the reject pile so it could be mine while I went through chemo. After all, I had repeatedly prayed that He put the right information into my hands. One reason we call Him Providence is because He inserts unexpected comforts into lives.

Yours Truly,

Lynette

Dear Leah,

Even though my cancer is gone, my digestion is now fine, my hair and my stamina have returned, my veins remember the trauma, my bones recall the pain, my stomach knows that nagging queasiness, and my brain has not forgotten how it was to dread and fear. As you endure your own treatment trauma, in the midst of it all, I urge you to practice thankfulness, because gratitude transforms what you do have even now. Articulating thankfulness for specific blessings will point out to you how wonderful it is to have them. Thankfulness can give a leisurely bath the feel of a spa or transform a drink into an oasis. Appreciation can even turn an attentive husband into "Prince Charming."

Our youth minister, Johnsie Henderson, recently asked this question, "If you could have nothing today that you had not uttered thanks to God for on yesterday, what would your life look like?" If you could posses no object, no talent, no friend, no gadget, nor any comfort except the ones you had recently spoken of to God, how different would your day be? That question made me want to be more observant and more specific. Often, especially while I was on chemo, I thanked God for clean sheets, the appliances to wash and dry them, for a pillow, a quiet bedroom, a hot water bottle, for soft covers, and the quilt made by my mama. Now is the time to take inventory. May God enable your eyes to see the blessings, your ears to hear the comforts, your heart to feel the encouragements, your brain to count the diversify. Yours Truly,

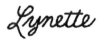

Dear Willadean,

I hope you had a nice birthday. It must have been extra special knowing that you are almost finished with chemo. I am so excited for you to be over this long ordeal. Today I have a story for you that is full of happiness, hope, healing, expectations, and appreciations.

In Luke 17, we are told of ten lepers who cry out for Jesus to heal them. Lepers were considered unclean and shameful. Jesus sees the ten and instructs them to show themselves to the priest. If a leper believed his disease was gone, he was to have a priest lift the quarantine and readmit him into society. As they are going, the ten are healed. Some might say healing was a coincidence or merely caused by time. Others may believe that their going earned their healing. However, one of the ten who is suddenly relieved of his leprosy recognizes it as Jesus' power and love. The man's faith causes him to return to Jesus with spontaneously personal appreciation. As this Samaritan glorifies God with a loud voice and falls on his face thanking Jesus, the Savior asks, "Were there not ten cleansed? But where are the nine?" (NKJV) The nine are doing what the Law of Moses required; they are religious but not whole-heartedly thankful. Jesus tells this singular man, "Arise, go your way. Your faith has made you well." (NKJV) The man's going has made him well. It has not earned him salvation, but it is obedient faith which puts him in the right relationship with Jesus to heal him.

True faith is never passive. Romans 16:25-26 discusses obedient faith. Regarding Jesus' statement, "Your faith has made you well," it could also be translated, "Your faith has saved you." My Bible's footnote tells me that the Greek word for "well" and "saved" are the same word. The Samaritan's faith does not even stop with complying. He takes time out from self-centered rejoicing and getting back to his loved ones when he changes directions and goes to thank the Giver. Why do the nine not return? Do they not see the healing as from Jesus? Do they prioritize the letter of the law over having a thankfully loving heart? Or, are they simply in a big hurry to get back to their normal lives as they had been before leprosy came?

For several years I have taught Bible classes of girls who are ages eight to eleven. During my nearly thirty years in the classroom, most behaviors I have seen repeated many times. However, there is one behavior I have rarely seen.

Not long ago I had a conscientious student named Caitlyn. Everyone was her friend and the feeling was mutual. Each week when class was over, as all the girls dashed out to play, to hang out with older friends, or to cuddle babies in the nursery, very often Caitlyn would lag behind just a minute for one purpose. She would walk to the door, change directions by turning back, sweetly smile and say, "Thank you for being my teacher." In my life of teaching, Caitlyn is not the one in ten; she is probably the one in 500. Of all the things I treasure about Caitlyn, that is the most unique. Her thankfulness showed me she counts her blessings and possesses perceptions and sympathy that compassionately cause her to imagine herself in the place of another person. Caitlyn's being willing to verbalize her appreciations showed me she was willing to delay her self-centered fun until after she took time to be thankful. Also, it showed me that she does not judge herself by the crowd. She did not decide to be like the majority and follow the flock to rush out the door. Finally, Caitlyn's thankfulness showed me that once is not enough for the thankful heart. I treasured each time Caitlyn spoke of her thanks, because each time it was fresh and from her heart.

As I completed my cancer treatments and as you are completing yours, there are many lessons to be absorbed from the story of the ten lepers:

(1) Even if a person's recovery is attributed to surgery, chemo, or radiation, in Acts 17:28, Paul says, "In Him we live and move and have our being." Recognize your life as initiated and sustained by God. He can use even doctors and medicines to accomplish His purposes.

(2) Real faith is not just mental and cannot be separated from action.

(3) The action does not earn salvation, but it gets one into the right relationship just as grabbing a life preserver when you are drowning. The grabbing does not earn the salvation for the drowning man, but he cannot be saved unless he grabs what God is extending.

(4) Do not always equate the outward look of religion with true appreciations.

(5) Thank the Giver even if it means changing your direction.

(6) Do not be in such a hurry to get back to your regular life that you do not take time to abundantly thank Jesus and also demonstrate your appreciations.

(7) Take time to be so lavish with fervent thankfulness that it praises God's glory and majesty.

You and I have so many things for which to be thankful!

Lynette

for further thought

1. When do we usually see God's fingerprints? Have you seen them?

2. Why can we not fathom all that God has done? (Ecclesiastes 3:11; Job 42:1-6; Romans 8:26-28)

3. What does it mean to "use adversity to stimulate you to creative survival?" (Luke 16:1-13)

4. Explain the statement, "Sometimes things happen in spite of all you or I do."

5. What are the negative and the positive of, "We cannot anticipate all the possibilities?" (James 4:13-16)

6. Analyze the poem "Answered Prayer."

7. How do you reconcile Acts 17:28 to the wonders of medicine or modern surgery?

8. Is faith in your mind, in your actions, or both? (Romans 16:25-26; Galatians 5:6; James 2:14-26)

9. Do your actions *earn* salvation? (Ephesians 2:8-10)

10. Does the outward look of religion guarantee that the heart is thankful? (Luke 18:9-14)

11. After prolonged illness, what is a possible pitfall of being in an extreme hurry to get back to your normal life?

12. Describe what lavish thankfulness does.

Chapter Twelve
Preventing or Thwarting Cancer

Songs

Purer Yet and Purer

We Are Called to Be God's People

Have You Counted the Cost?

Dare to Be a Daniel

My Jesus, I Love Thee

What Would Jesus Do?

O Be Careful Little Hands What You Do

Open My Eyes That I May See

Purer in Heart, O God

More Love to Thee O Christ

Savior, Teach Me, Day By Day

Guide Me O Thou Great Jehovah

My Life, My Love I Give to Thee

O **Great Physician,** Encourage me to seek **knowledge** and **wisdom** as sent by You but not use it as a **substitute** for You.

Depending on your history and individual needs, with this chapter I hope to:

(1) Reduce your risk of getting cancer by: fortifying your immune system, ridding your body of cancer-causing substances, and thwarting processes that contribute to cancer formation;

(2) Strengthen bodies for whom treatment brought weakness or caused muscle atrophy;

(3) Lower the risk of recurrent cancer;

(4) Starve or slow down the growth of any cancer you may still have;

(5) Give you new vigor, stamina, health, and improve your mental outlook.

Prevention is always better than cure. If you have had cancer, chances are that now you are being regularly tested for the return of the cancer you had or for certain related cancers. It is wise to research these tests to understand their validity and meanings. However, do not let having tests lull you into thinking you can ignore unhealthy foods or an unsound lifestyle. Most tests do not keep one from getting cancer but are for the purpose of catching cancer early. Prevention is still better. You are the conductor of this symphony to save your life. Your orchestration should be a harmony of particular lifestyle changes including offense and defense. It was because of my not being able to follow the usual plan for cancer patients in my circumstances that I began intensive research into what to do naturally that would thwart the return of cancer or eliminate any new cancer.

Current scientific literature credits our environment with causing approximately 80% of cancers, while 10-20% are believed to be hereditary. However, even hereditary cancers may be accelerated or abated by one's lifestyle. Since I do not believe my cancer was hereditary, my lifestyle, environment, or a pharmaceutical caused my cancer. Because of that, I will not keep doing all the exact same things I had been doing. For example, never again will I take hormone replacement therapy. I should not feel guilty for making what I believed at the time to be the best choices. However, now we have more information, therefore there are additional things I now do to diminish my risks of cancer. I encourage you to not wait for a medical mandate, a nation-wide alert, or a smoking gun of any type. Research on your own what could extend your future, your quality of life, and that of your family.

Excitedly I read about a variety of lifestyle changes that can *each* slightly reduce one's risk of cancer. In addition, these precautions simultaneously reduce risks of heart attack, stroke, arthritis, high blood pressure, cholesterol, diabetes, and osteoporosis. A plethora of scientific studies are now underway to give us more information about specific foods, supplements, exercise, and avoidances that can make us healthier people. Because of my hyper-sensitivities to pharmaceuticals, I chose the natural method.

The scrutinizing which each normal cell does can be compared to a computer's spell-checker. Many times each day cells are hit by toxins. Your body looks for trouble, but the efficiency of this proofreading system declines with each advancing decade, and more errors evade the spell-checker. If the repair crew gets weak or cells are made too fast, cancer may begin. A cancer cell clones itself. This mass can become a tumor which endeavors to hide, feed, and spread. It tries to elude the immune system's surveillance, set up a blood supply through the process of angiogenesis, and colonize in distant tissue through metastasis. According to Dr. Bob Arnot, autopsies performed on women in their forties reveal that 40% who died of causes unrelated to cancer already had tiny breast malignancies. A tumor must have a billion cells for mammography to detect it. Begin today enhancing your natural defenses.

Nutritional information is constantly being updated, but current recommendations are:

(1) Take NO supplements while on chemo, unless your oncologist approves. These can contradict chemo.

(2) Study nutrition from various sources with different philosophies. Weigh their credibility.

(3) Read information that is very current and that relies on scientific studies, not just testimonials.

(4) Read information that is from different types of sources, not just books or not only from the Internet.

(5) Learn some of the jargon of the profession of nutritional science to understand the literature.

(6) Take notes or make copies of information that pertains to you and any illness for which you are at risk.

(7) Be aware of precautions concerning taking herbs or supplements. Some interfere with other drugs by negating or exaggerating their effects. Complete precautions will *not* be listed on a supplement's bottle. Write down the names and amounts of each one you want to take. If you are on any prescription, get your doctor's approval to begin a supplement. Wait four days to add any other new supplement.

(8) Keep a thorough food and drink diary for a week. Look for deficiencies or excesses. Choose a nutritionist who specializes in your health needs. Have her evaluate your food diary. Ask her questions.

(9) Discuss nutrition with investigative people who have or had the same type cancer as you.

(10) Collect articles such as from *The American Institute of Cancer Research* at 1 (800) 843-8114.

Several years ago while at the University of Tennessee, I heard three students talking. The young man said he had taken a multi-vitamin and mineral supplement the previous evening and could not sleep. He asked friends if they thought that it could be the pill that kept him awake. They thought that was a ridiculous idea. Since that time, I too have had the experience of some supplements keeping me awake. When I advise that you investigate any substance before you take it, even research what time of day you should take each particular supplement or if there could be conflicts. For example, iron should not be taken with calcium. Most supplements should be taken with a meal, but a few should be taken on an empty stomach. Some supplements should not be taken in the evening. However, melatonin is meant to be taken at night. Investigation is paramount.

LIFESTYLE HABITS THAT REPORTEDLY *INCREASE* ONE'S RISK OF GETTING CANCER:

    smoking or living with passive smoke,

    drinking alcohol,

    obesity,

    daily eating meats, especially meats that are smoked, charcoal broiled or have nitrates or nitrites,

    an abundance of omega-6 fatty acids from margarine or oils,

regularly eating white bread, white rice, white pasta, and bleached white flour,

eating fewer than four fruits and vegetables daily,

more than five ounces of sugar daily (including in beverages),

a diet high in salt and low in potassium, and

exposure to electromagnetic fields, radiation, or emissions (Example: telephone lineman).

Women have the added increased risk of breast cancer from:

hormone replacement therapy, oral contraceptives,

having had no biological children, having had the first child after age thirty, and having not breast fed for at least three months.

LIFESTYLE HABITS THAT REPORTEDLY *REDUCE* ONES CHANCES OF GETTING CANCER:

taking a multi-vitamin/mineral that includes folic acid and sufficient antioxidants,

regular exercise,

eating five to ten fruits and vegetables daily,

eating cold water fish or taking a "clean" fish oil supplement,

often eating cruciferous vegetables such as broccoli, often eating beans,

eating garlic and olive oil, eating whole grains daily,

eating yogurt or buttermilk with lactobacillus acidophilus and bifidobacterium bifidum,

drinking green tea daily, and at least 2.5 liters of water.

These lifestyle risk factors are not prioritized. Adopting one factor that *reduces* cancer's risk does not exactly negate the effects of one factor that *increases* the risk of cancer. I discuss only factors you can modify. Other research can address such risks as age or genetics. Also, I will not debate the soy issue because: (1) For those whose cancer was estrogen receptive, soy is off limits, (2) its benefits to specific individuals is controversial, (3) measuring how much effective soy is in various foods and brands is extremely confusing. However, if you had estrogen receptive cancer and are avoiding soy, also avoid lima beans and garbanzo beans (chickpeas). Yes, soy seems to benefit those who have never had cancer, but we still need large controlled scientific studies of how soy effects those who have had an estrogen receptive tumor. According to the American Institute of Cancer Research, a researcher experimenting with genistein found in soy discovered that it works ten times better in discouraging cancer growth in noncancerous cells than in cells where cancer growth had already started.

Doctors do not know all the latest in nutrition. Although a nutritionist can know the most current facts, she may not know ramifications of your medical history. Likewise, *I cannot recommend that you eat certain foods or supplements. Each person is different, so learn your own needs and restrictions.* Nutritional information is rapidly changing. I recommend using several sources in print, in person, and the Internet to *research* these habits.

Using tobacco or alcohol is a detriment to your health in many ways. There are so many well publicized negative things to say about each habit that I will not attempt to restate what we have already been told many times. However, you may not know that alcohol robs the body of nutrients, diminishes one's ability to destroy free radicals, and inactivates enzymes that repair damaged genes. It is also worth mentioning that 15% of people who get lung cancer have never smoked, but often these individuals were exposed to passive smoke. For people who are in a smoke-filled environment, a diet rich in carotenes and antioxidants is especially important. Carotene supplementation does not seem to work. It can even contribute to lung and colon cancer. Over supplementing with one carotenoid may keep the body from absorbing other carotenoids. The *Archives of Internal Medicine* reports that recently four physicians have discovered a previously unreported early warning sign for lung cancer. If you notice food suddenly tasting unpleasantly sweet, quickly tell your doctor. Apparently, a lung tumor causes the secretion of a hormone which distorts the ability of taste receptors in the tongue.

Obesity increases one's risk for several types of cancer. Weight that is 20% above the recommended pounds for your height is obesity. One of the most potent weapons against cancer is your fork and all that it holds or does not hold. Your odds improve or worsen with every bite. According to the *Medical Tribune*, waist size is an indication of internal abdominal fat which for a man can be pressing on his prostate, eventually resulting in urinary obstruction. A Harvard study of 50,000 men showed that men who gain more than forty pounds after age twenty-one are twice as likely to develop colon cancer. The *Journal of the American Medical Association* reports that post menopausal women who have gained more than forty-four pounds since age eighteen are twice as likely to develop breast cancer. Relatively heavy women over fifty who gained more than ten pounds since their forties triple their risk. Visceral fat causes a cascade of negative metabolic effects.

Exercising works. While I understood the benefits exercise has against heart disease or osteoporosis, I was flabbergasted to read that lack of exercise is a risk factor for developing cancers. In scientific studies conducted at Harvard, if a woman had been a college athlete, her risk for tumors of the uterus, ovaries, cervix, vagina, and breast was reduced by 50-70% over women who had not exercised regularly. Exercise reduces a woman's estrogen production, stimulates its inactivation, diminishes abdominal fat, and reduces insulin. Estrogen that is not metabolized or excreted can linger in the body, become aggressive, and cause cells to divide faster. Cells which divide faster may duplicate into a flawed cell that turns cancerous. Exercise also helps one sweat which eliminates toxins. Include drinking more water. The skin is sometimes even called the "third kidney."

Eat 5-10 servings of fruits and vegetables every day. Fruits and vegetables have been called the natural pharmacy. They contain hundreds of known and unknown phytochemicals which benefit our bodies in ways we do not always understand. Yet only 11% of Americans follow this recommendation. In addition, fruits and vegetables provide benefits not available in supplements. These phytochemicals have a synergistic effect with other vitamins, minerals, or phytochemicals that cannot be achieved without eating the fruit or vegetable. The National Cancer Institute reviewed 200 published scientific reports and found that all organs of the body can have their cancer rates cut in half or even more by eating an abundance of fruits and vegetables. Bright or dark fruits and vegetables are especially rich in phytochemicals such as carotenes (found in carrots, spinach, tomatoes, and sweet potatoes) and flavonoids (found in berries and citrus) These work in harmony with antioxidants such as vitamins C, E, and selenium, but phytochemicals are now believed to be just as important in the fight against cancer. Findings at the University of California showed that when supplemental pills challenge natural food, foods often far surpass the tablets. A food with 10 I.U. of vitamin E silenced as many free radicals as 800 I.U. of vitamin E from a pill, and 60 mg. of vitamin C from food was equal to 800 mg. of vitamin C in a supplement.

In a March 2003 study, scientists report that organically grown corn and strawberries show significantly higher levels of cancer-fighting antioxidants than conventionally grown foods. It seems that pesticides and herbicides thwart the production of phenolics which act as a plant's natural defense and contribute to good health.

Tufts University has ranked fruits and vegetables into three groups depending upon their scores in antioxidant potential. They named this ranking the ORAC scores. (Oxygen Radical Absorbence Capacity.) Those in Group One contain the highest levels of antioxidants and include such foods as: garlic, kale, spinach, broccoli, brussels sprouts, beets, strawberries, plums, prunes, Concord grapes, blueberries, and blackberries. However, scientists recommend eating three from each group daily which would total nine fruits and vegetables. To best protect your natural defenses against all cancers, Laura Pawlak PhD, RD recommends these foods: broccoli, carrot, tomato, strawberries, green tea, garlic, flax seeds, wheat germ, tangerines and oranges. (People taking a prescription blood thinner cannot eat foods high in Vitamin K unless their doctor adjusts their dosage.)

If you are targeting your fight against a specific cancer, often eat these plants. For those wishing to thwart breast cancer, the recommended foods are: tangerine, broccoli, wheat germ, olive oil, avocado, green tea, and flax seeds. Tufts University states that concerning breast cancer, the combination of natural chemicals in a tangerine is 5 to 250 times more powerful against that specific cancer than the genistein in soy which had been reported to have such promise! For those wanting to specifically prevent prostate cancer, often choose: tomatoes (especially cooked), melons, cucumbers, squash, pumpkin seeds, and cold water fish. To diminish chances of lung cancer, often eat: strawberries, tangerines, oranges, carrots, guava, tomatoes, V-8 cocktail juice, and green tea. Broccoli contains phytochemicals which trigger the formation of GST, the enzyme which carts away carcinogens, notably those in cigarette smoke. Broccoli sprouts have very concentrated isothiocyanates and extra cancer protection. (Wash thoroughly.) Daily eat a cruciferous vegetable or, for when you cannot, ask your doctor about taking an indole-3 supplement. Avoid eating antacids with cruciferous vegetables.

Produce grown in foreign countries is more likely to contain pesticides banned in the U. S. Even U.S. strawberries, apples, and peaches are notorious for residual pesticides or herbicides, yet do not avoid produce and its benefits. Your choices are: grow your own, buy from a local person who limits possible hazards, or use an organic grocer, plus throughly wash produce in an all-natural food cleanser available at health food stores.

Eat more fiber. Gastroenterologists and Sloan-Kettering's Comprehensive Breast Center recommend 25-30g daily. Dr. Bob Arnot recommends 30-50g. Most Americans eat 12g. The cellulose and pectin in fiber show anti-cancer activity. The fiber in whole grains is also rich in vitamin E which enhances the immune system, decreases mutations, and aids membrane resilience. When baking, try replacing a fraction of the flour with wheat germ, or sprinkle wheat germ on oatmeal or yogurt. A half-ounce of wheat bran can reduce bile acids in the colon by half. Chronic constipation is a risk factor for breast cancer and colon cancer. It is the function of the intestines and the kidneys to dispose of excess estrogen. Women excrete a large percentage of the body's estrogen in their bowel movements. If the contents of your digestive system linger in your body, intestinal estrogen will be reabsorbed. In contrast, fiber escorts estrogen out faster so it is not reabsorbed into the blood through pores in the colon wall. Reabsorbed estrogen is aggressive. If greater amounts of intestinal estrogen are being eliminated, there will be less risk of cells that are made speedily and incorrectly. See relevant studies conducted at the Tufts New England Medical Center regarding fiber. (If you are post menopausal, do not assume you have no estrogen. When ovaries decline in estrogen production, fat cells and the adrenal gland still make it.) Gradually begin any fiber increase. Your body will slowly adjust. Again, include drinking eight to ten glasses of water each day.

Eat more nuts. (Store all nuts in the refrigerator or freezer.) Choose nuts that are dry roasted and not coated. The nut should be the only ingredient. Walnuts and pecans, (along with strawberries, raspberries, grapes, apples, and pomegranates) contain ellagic acid which scavengers for carcinogens. In animal studies ellagic acid inhibited tumor growth from esophageal cancer. Look for research in the journal *Carcinogenesis*. Ellagic acid is not available in supplement form. Walnuts also contain the good Omega-3 fatty acid and Co-Q-10.

Change to organic beef. Unlike most beef, organic beef contains no growth hormones, antibiotics, or pesticides. In forty-four states, organic beef is sold under the name Laura's Lean. This beef has the approval of the American Heart Association. It can also be investigated at www.laurasleanbeef.com or by calling 1-800-ITS-LEAN. I have found Laura's Lean ground beef to keep longer in the refrigerator, have less fat, brown faster, and have a wonderful taste. Although Laura's Lean is in many cities, for those west of the Mississippi River, sometimes the Maverick Ranch brand organic beef may be more available.

Change to organic milk, yogurt, and cheese. Brands to look for are: Horizon, Organic Valley, Stonyfield, or Naturally Preferred. One would think it is advisable to get the no-fat varieties, however, Conjugated Linoleic Acid (CLA) is found in dairy fat and is reported to fight cancer. (Investigate current data on CLA.) I usually get organic milk with 1% fat content. Using organic skim milk in the dry form is a clever way to fortify baking or mashed potatoes with an extra amount of milk. When I mix up the dry ingredients for pancakes or breads, I stir in milk powder. That allows it to dissolve better than adding it to liquid. Large amounts of organic dry milk can be ordered from Organic Valley at 1 (888) 444-6455. You and a friend could order together.

Avoid nitrates and nitrites. These are found in lunch meats, wieners, pastrami, and bacon. A couple of brands of roasted turkey breast do not contain nitrates or nitrites. Read labels. According to Dr. Michael Murray, children who eat three hot dogs per week have ten times the risk of developing leukemia compared to those who do not eat hot dogs. If you eat meats with nitrates or nitrites, increase your vitamin C intake.

Meat gives us iron, protein and B vitamins, but in general, nutritionists recommend that Americans decrease the times per week they eat meat and reduce each portion to three ounces or less (the size of a deck of cards). Cut away any fat you see, and drain ground beef very well. Precautions usually include these facts: high fat diets suppress the immune system; contribute to many health problems; require a body work extra hard to metabolize animal fat, and the process can produce free radicals; plus, animal fat holds environmental toxins longer than plant fats. Diets high in meat raise the risk of all kinds of cancer. Meat fat causes a body to secrete extra bile acids to digest it. Bile acids are thought to contribute to colon cancer. According the National Cancer Institute, people who eat large amounts of red meat double their risk of non-Hodgkin's lymphoma. The manner in which meat is prepared also affects its ability to cause cancer. Meat that is fried, charcoaled, smoked, or overly cooked at high temperatures is more likely to cause cancer, because heterocyclic amines are brought out.

Avoid bad fats and increase good fats. Saturated fats such as meat fat, lard, or coconut oil are bad fats. These may also be hidden in crackers, cookies, chips, gravy, and fast foods. When the intake of bad fat is high, tumors are more likely to metastasize. Recently the National Institute of Medicine declared that NO amount of trans-fatty acids, as found in margarine and some snacks is safe. Hydrogenated or partially hydrogenated oils also have omega-**6** fatty acid and are being shown to do detriment to the body. Americans eat far too much of the omega-6 oils found in meats, margarine, and most vegetable oils. They usually have a deficiency of omega-**3** fatty acids found in cold water fish or flaxseed. Bodies require a balance between omega-6 and omega-3. A diet that includes large amounts of saturated fats, cholesterol, and margarine makes cell membranes that lose their ability to communicate with other cells or to hold nutrients, thus cells are injured. Cell membrane dysfunction is often the beginning of cancer. American diets contain 20-500 times too much omega-6. Nutritionists recommend cold water fish rich in omega-3, but the specific fish recommended varies from one nutritionist to another, except they all recommend avoiding swordfish and shark. Norway seems to be the primary source of pollution-free fish for making the fish oil supplements found in health food stores, and there they are also raising salmon in pollution-free fjords. The Comprehensive Breast Cancer Centers at Sloan-Kettering and UCLA recommend 2 - 10g of daily fish oil supplement, depending on your history. Choose brands that are molecularly distilled or steam-stripped to remove toxins. The work of Dr. John Glaspy shows only three months of fish oils can change the composition of the breasts and make them more resistant to cancer. Besides omega-6 and omega-3, there is omega-**9** as found in olive oil and canola oil. Diets rich in olive oil seem to promote health, possibly because these diets are lower in omega-6. Substitutions can be made for foods high in omega-6. *Depending on the recipe*, possible alternatives for mayonnaise, margarine, and shortening include: yogurt, applesauce, prune puree, olive oil, or canola oil. The measurements and the cooking temperature may have to be adjusted. Poultry farmers who raise hens for Eggland's brand eggs feed their chickens a diet that produces eggs with less saturated fat and more omega-3.

Avoid adding salt pit type salt. A high-sodium and low-potassium diet can increase the risk of esophageal and colon cancers. Nutritionists recommend sea salt or the substitutes Nu-Salt or NoSalt. Try flavoring more with spices, herbs, and lemon juice instead of salt. If you gradually decrease your use of salt, you will not feel so deprived, and your taste buds will adjust.

Avoid or limit Hormone Replacement Therapy Limit any additional exposure to estrogen, even if the source is natural or prescribed. Of eighteen known risk factors for breast cancer, at least fourteen are connected to increases in estrogen. For example, being an older woman, being obese, not exercising, and having had no children each increases the risks for developing breast cancer because each factor has given a woman added exposure to estrogen. However, not every risk has the same weight. Reportedly, HRT is one of the risk factors with a heavier weight—more likely to put you in jeopardy. HRT has recently been shown to not protect the heart, and there are natural means of thwarting osteoporosis. I have been shocked by the cavalier attitude of some medical people over recommending HRT to their patients. Weigh all advice and research on your own.

Avoid heating foods in plastic. Never microwave in a plastic container or in plastic wrap. This process disperses plastic particles into food! Glass is the safest microwave container, if it passes this test. Microwave an empty glass container one minute. If it is cool, use it for microwaving. If it is warm, do not.

Avoid tanning beds. *The New England Journal of Medicine* says no span of time in a tanning bed is safe.

Reduce the amount of processed sugar used. Sugar is most damaging when eaten or drunk on an empty stomach. Both sugar and insulin released to process it speed the growth of cancers. Excessive sugar has been shown to decrease the immune system. Try smaller portions, reduce sugar in recipes, and drink beverages with no added sugar. When evaluating the amount of sugar you eat, do not forget to count your sugared drinks. The average American daily eats and drinks six times the amount of sugar he should have.

Limit artificially colored foods and preservatives. I use gelatin with no added colors and no sugar. First dissolve it in a small amount of cold water, and then put that into boiling water. I choose brands of fruit pie-filling with no added dyes and canned vegetables with no preservatives. Whether a food is bought in a grocery chain or at a health foods store, discover which brands do not use ingredients you should avoid. To specifically prevent pancreatic cancer, the avoidance of preservatives, additives, or grilling is especially important.

Limit exposure to permanent hair colors. People who regularly use permanent hair colors are reported to eventually double their chances of bladder cancer. With the accumulation of years, cosmetologists are at five times higher risk for bladder cancer. Temporary hair coloring has not been shown to have this risk.

Limit exposure to hazardous chemicals. Investigate the solvents and cleaning products you use. Minimize exposure to noxious fumes even from gasoline, glues, varnish, and fingernail polish remover. Change to a more user friendly detergent or add one cup of white vinegar in the final rinse. Limit use of fabric softener.

Limit caffeine. Caffeine is believed to cause an increase in insulin that retards the burning of stored fat. Excessive caffeine thwarts DNA repair and is linked to urinary cancer. People who drink more than four cups of coffee daily are four times as likely to develop colon cancer. Human studies also show that daily eating a chocolate bar doubles colon cancer's risk. See *Journal of the National Cancer Institute* and *Mutation Research*.

Bromelain Enzyme is found in FRESH pineapples and kiwi. It is what will not let gelatin congeal if it contains fresh forms of these fruits. Studies in Germany have found that a bromelain supplement stimulates immune function and prevent platelets from sticking together. Sometimes bromelain is prescribed along with papaya enzyme. These should be taken with meals if they are enteric coated. If not coated with a layer that will not be dissolved by stomach juices, then they should be taken on an empty stomach. In the past, scientists have said that enzyme supplements would not be absorbed. However, according to Drs. Michael Murray and Tim Birdsall, recent research has shown that enzymes taken orally are absorbed intact. See "Cancer Patients Should Eat Pineapple" from the *International Journal of Alternative and Complimentary Medicine*. Research and ask your doctor. Do not take Bromelain if you are on an anti-coagulant or if you have high blood pressure.

Co-Q-10 The body uses this coenzyme as an antioxidant. It stimulates the immune system and is in salmon, peanuts, walnuts, and spinach. Deficient levels of Co-Q-10 have been found in patients with cancers of the lung, breast, prostate, pancreas, colon, kidney, and brain as well as those with myeloma and lymphoma. Some oncologists recommend it be taken during specifically scheduled days of chemotherapy to prevent damage that can be caused by Adriamycin or Methotrexate. On other days it must be avoided so that chemo can do its work. While on chemo, let your oncologist schedule days you will take it and days you will abstain. In one study among patients who had either breast cancer or prostate cancer, deaths were significantly lower among those who took Co-Q-10 supplements. See the National Cancer Institute web site http://nccam.nih.gov or call: 1 (888) 644-6226. Investigate studies in *Biochemical and Biophysical Research Communications* and in *Molecular Aspects of Medicine*. Co-Q-10 may alter the body's response to anti-coagulants or insulin.

Green Tea is like the tea we regularly drink except it is unfermented, and it has more phytochemicals. Green tea is the only food to contain the polyphenol EGCG which is one of the most potent antioxidants yet discovered. These compounds appear to aid the immune system, prevent angiogenesis, thwart metastasis, lower cholesterol, and protect against various cancers. Increased consumption of green tea is correlated to decreased reoccurrence of breast cancer. Steep your own; bottled tea is not as nutritious. It also comes decaffeinated.

Flax Seeds This unusual food is rich in omega-3 fatty acids, such as Alpha Linolenic Acid (ALA), and it is rich in lignans which act as an anti-estrogen. According to Dr. Michael Murray, these interfere with the cancer-promoting effects of estrogen on breast tissue. Lignans also increase the production of Sex Hormone Binding Globulin (SHBG). This protein escorts estrogen out of the body. In the lab flax seeds thwarted colon cancer and skin cancer, reduced breast tumors, and prevented metastasis. Murray recommends freshly ground flaxseed to prevent or treat prostate cancer. However, he suggests that flaxseed *oil* be avoided by men who currently have prostate cancer. In a study conducted at Duke University and Veterans Medical Center involving men with prostate cancer, a low fat diet that included two tablespoons of freshly ground flax seed slowed cancer growth. Flaxseeds must be kept in the refrigerator. Immediately before use, I chop mine in a small coffee grinder. Flax seeds work best when mixed with sulfur-rich protein foods such as low-fat cottage cheese, beans, or peas. It can be ordered from Heintzmann Farms at 1-800-333-5813. Look for articles in the *Journal of Nutrition*. Avoid flax seeds if you have inflammatory disease of the esophagus, stomach, or intestine. Discuss flax with you doctor.

Melatonin This is a substance made in the brain's pineal gland, but with age, the amount made diminishes. Russel Reiter of the University of Texas Health Science Center has researched melatonin for thirty-five years. Other research is spread throughout journals in the fields of oncology, cardiology, gerontology, chronobiology, and immunology. This variety of data has shown melatonin boosts the immune system, protects against some environmental hazards, gives anti-oxidant protection, lowers cholesterol, normalizes blood pressure, relieves depression, remedies jet lag, and promotes normal sleep. For thousands with terminal cancer, it has been shown to prolong the survival and improve quality of life. Look for research in *Lancet, The Journal of Pineal Research, Journal of Neural Transmission, British Journal of Cancer*, and the *Annals of the New York Academy of Science*. There are studies showing melatonin inhibiting prostate cancer and breast cancer. Controlled studies show melatonin alone is usually no magic bullet, but when combined with other treatments, it allows patients to live longer and have better quality of life than the surgery or treatments without melatonin. Investigate these studies for yourself, keeping in mind that the reason for taking the melatonin will determine the dosage. Many people take a fraction of a milligram (0.2 to 1mg). Investing in a pill splitter may be a good idea. Your research and doctor can help you know whether to take it and at what dosage. Since melatonin is to be taken at bedtime, choose a supplement that contains no vitamins which might keep you awake. If it makes you have wild dreams, try a different manufacturer or a lower dosage. For ten per cent of the population melatonin supplements have the opposite affect and will keep them awake. It has never been shown to be toxic.

Coral Calcium Plus See www.bodygenix.com or call: 1-877-643-9853. Coral Calcium can also be purchased at discount stores and pharmacies. *The Journal of the American Medical Association* reports that increasing calcium can help prevent cancer of the pancreas, prostate, colon, and breast. Calcium is involved in: electrical energy for heart beat, all muscle responses, DNA replication, and feeding every cell. It boosts the immune system, breaks down heavy metals and residues, strengthens tissue, increases mobility, combats arthritis, heart disease, digestive problems, cholesterol, osteo-porosis, and cataracts. When my chemo was over, I tried various types, brands, and forms of calcium and *tripled* the amount of milk I was drinking, hoping to diminish my bone pain, but I felt no relief. I was still praying for the right people and the correct information to come into my life. For ten months I studied and tried a variety of natural substances. None relieved my bone pain. When my sister-in-law told me that pharmacist Mark Binkley suggested she investigate Coral Calcium, I asked my rheumatologist for per-mission to try it. He would not prescribe me any pharmaceutical, but gave me his blessing to begin Coral Calcium. My improvements were sudden and fantastically noticeable to me, my family, to Laura Weisberg my wonderful physical therapist, and my friends. After I had such great results with this form of calcium, I told my friend Barbara about it. She has fibromyalgia and has also tried various forms of calcium. In a few days each would make her sick. However, Coral Calcium has also worked great for Barbara. Coral Calcium contains magnesium, trace minerals, and Vitamin D and is ionized. When I began taking the capsules, I discovered that taking one at night made my mind too energetic to sleep. I take one each morning and continue to eat and drink calcium rich foods. Harvesting Coral Calcium does not harm the environment. Regarding hype that surrounds advertising for Coral Calcium, I am neither discouraged nor overly impressed by it. My investigations con-cerning calcium focus on renowned scientific information. Although I tried to get bone pain relief from foods and various calcium supplements, it was Coral Calcium *alone* that quickly improved my quality of living in many ways.

Vitamin D. Countries with more sunlight often have fewer cases of breast cancer. Sunlight helps bodies make Vitamin D. A recent Massachusetts study showed 59% of hospital patients had Vitamin D defi-ciencies. Get five minutes of rays when the sun is not at peak intensity. Fortified milk and Coral Calcium also have Vitamin D.

Aspirin are reported to thwart cancers of the esophagus and colon. Taking many aspirin can damage the stomach, but due to the Nurses' Health Study, gastroenerologists recommend one aspirin three times a week.

Read labels. Evaluate the type and amount of fat, assess the sugar content, and avoid dyes or nitrite.

Treat ulcers or chronic heartburn. Ulcers may eventually put a person at risk for stomach cancer. Blood tests can tell if Helicobacter pylori bacteria caused an ulcer. The remedy is antibiotics and bismuth subsalicylate. In two weeks the risk of stomach cancer will be lowered. Reflux of stomach acid is a known risk factor for esophageal cancer. Heartburn sufferers, do not eat near bedtime, stay upright soon after a meal, lose weight, wear loose clothes, and avoid coffee, alcohol, fat, spices, peppermint, and chocolate.

Slowly modify recipes, diet, supplements, or lifestyle. This increases your ability to maintain reform. No precaution, food, avoidance, or supplement I have listed is the one magic answer for all people to inhibit cancer, but possibly together these can be that symphony to save your life. In addition, they will help a person feel more energetic. As more scientific studies are concluded, there may be substances now unheard of that will be shown to thwart cancer. Keep researching. Consult your doctor, but do not depend on any physician to be knowledgeable concerning all the current findings in nutrition. Of course, he or she will know some information, but it is more than a medical doctor can read to stay current in both his field and the field of nutrition. The National Cancer Institute has a toll-free telephone number. They have nutritionists who answer questions at: 1-800-4-CANCER or 1-800-422-6237. The American Dietetic Association will also answer questions at: 1-800-366-1655. To speak personally with a dietician call Dial-A-Dietician at: 1-900-CALL-AN-RD. You can discuss your concerns for the cost of $1.95 for the first minute and then $.95 per minute after that. (Timing begins when questions begin.) Nutritionists do not all have the same level of expertise, interest, and specialty. I have discussed diet with four nutritionists and seen a wide difference among them. If one does not fit your needs, find another. The knowledgeable nutritionists I have relied upon most often are Dr. Autumn Chester Marshall at Lipscomb University and Dr. Mary Sue Walker who volunteers at Knoxville's Wellness Community. Several years ago, Mary Sue's brother was diagnosed with colon cancer. He was a dentist and therefore already had a scientific background, but to treat himself, he chose to use a very extreme diet. Mary Sue saw her brother deteriorate and his cancer became aggravated. She believes that nutritional mis-information contributed to his death. Yes, he had read and studied, but it was only from one point of view. Mary Sue resolved to get her PhD in nutrition in order to not only advise cancer patients, but also to be able to explain the reasoning behind her advice.

I urge you to get a nutrition partner who is investigative. Because she will use different libraries, periodicals, or Internet sites, she will have information you do not, and you will discover information she does not. It is more fun when you can each feel you are helping keep the other cancer-free. My sister-in-law and I did this by e-mail. We traded not only facts but also names and addresses of where to find more information.

During all your research that may be both depressing and reassuring, I encourage you to laugh, play and feel joy. Sprinkle your life with the comics, joke books, video comedies, funny cassettes, witty friends, and sweet children. Do not let anyone rob you of your hope.

Dear Edd,

It is wonderful that you are off the medicine which wrecked your stamina. When I finished chemo and could not tolerate drug therapy, I tried various foods and supplements to ease bone pain. Then I abandoned any supplement that did not improve me or did not have documented scientific evidence of its ability to inhibit cancer. Through all this, my bone pain never subsided. I went from doctor to doctor but none helped me. Upon the recommendation of a pharmacist, I began taking Coral Calcium Plus in January 2002. In three days I started feeling better, and the difference in two weeks was remarkable. All at once people began telling me specifically how I looked better. My physical therapist told me my muscles were suddenly working better, my eyes were brighter, my skin color improved. I smiled much more, and I began often singing. My bone pain diminished, my outlook improved, I slept better, and could remember more. If your oncologist approves of the Coral Calcium and you want to possibly feel drastically better, try it for a month. Don't say, "Well, I have taken calcium before." This is like no other calcium! I believe that the cancer drugs you and I took depleted our bodies in dozens of ways. These minerals in the capsule can help us get back to optimal health and feeling drastically better!

Anticipating your recovery,

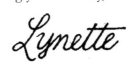

Dear Willadean,

As you rejoin the hubbub of life, unlike some uninformed individuals, do not put demands on your body too soon. Remember that your body has been through a trauma, and thus you are going to need to give it time to readjust and heal. Notice each improvement and thank God. Help your body get stronger by doing these things:

(1) Take a multi-vitamin/mineral supplement.

(2) Read about nutrition.

(3) Eat more fruits and vegetables that inhibit cancer.

(4) Gradually begin walking or some other exercise that can become an aerobic workout.

(5) Gradually begin a few upper body exercises to get back muscle you probably lost. These can be enhanced by lifting free-weights. I began by lifting a can of tuna in each hand, then cans of soup, then one pound weights. I also used a stretchy band looped around a door knob. Pulling on it can build arm and shoulder muscles. A physical therapist taught me how to do these exercises. If you point out to your doctor that your muscles have weakened, he can refer you to the physical therapist so that insurance will pay for it. ASK.

(6) Set aside a time for an afternoon nap or a rest period. Smile.

Love,

Lynette

Books, television, the Internet, and word of mouth led me to many valued discoveries. Even though they are each like a precious jewel to me, making me feel that these strategies could accumulatively keep cancer away from my future, I must still not let them become my "chariot." I find out all the information that I can, but knowing that it is God, not science, I must look to for my strength and real security.

1. Does a person's diet and lifestyle contribute to his either being healthy or unhealthy?

2. Why should you use various sources when you investigate health or nutrition?

3. Using Daniel 1:1-20, what types of foods would have made up a royal table?

4. What do we see that Daniel knew about royal foods versus a diet of vegetables and water?

5. If your diet includes lots of meats, bad fats, or many sweets, which of these two diets does it resemble?

6. Explain the meaning of Romans 12:1-2.

7. Discuss Biblical admonitions against gluttony (Proverbs 23:20-21) and for self-control (Galatians 5:23; II Peter 1:5-7).

8. If a Christian is to not pattern himself after the world, and if he is to be as a pilgrim, stranger, or alien on this earth (I Peter 2:9-12), then we accept that his speech, actions, and dress will sometimes be a contrast to the world's. How might what he eats and drinks also differ from what the world consumes?

9. Why did God implement dietary laws in the Old Testament?

10. Books, bracelets, and T-shirts have asked, "What would Jesus do?" There is now a book entitled. *What Would Jesus Eat?* What did Jesus eat? What would He eat today?

Chapter Thirteen
Becoming a Better Comforter

Songs

I Want to Be More Like Jesus

Bind Us Together

Each Day I'll Do a Golden Deed

O To Be Like Thee

In My Life Lord, Be Glorified

Is Your Life a Channel of Blessings?

To Love Someone More Dearly Every Day

Let the Beauty of Jesus Be Seen in Me

Lord, Make Us Instruments

A Charge to Keep I Have

There is a Sea

Rise Up O Men of God

Love One Another

Servant Song

I'll Live For Him

Lord, as You comforted me in a myriad of ways, help me to comfort others.

At the end of treatments, a person may be so anxious to put these struggles in the past that he or she tries to resume life just as it was before cancer made itself known. In contrast, I took the cancer announcement as a warning alarm. Even though I had always eaten a healthy diet, I wanted to increase my efforts toward prevention. Physically, I wanted to make the experience matter. However, beyond the new physical precautions I was beginning, spiritually I also wanted to make the cancer experience matter. When God looks at me now, I do not want Him to see me spiritually weakened nor spiritually walking in place, getting nowhere. Instead, I want Him to see that by leaning on Him, the struggles have strengthened me both within and without.

During a question and answer period after a lecture on mental health, Dr. Karl Menninger, the famous psychiatrist, was asked what he would advise a person to do if he or she felt a nervous breakdown coming on. Most people would expect him to stress going to a psychiatrist. To their astonishment, Dr. Menninger said, "Find somebody in need, and help that person."

Dear Chris,

Many years ago, our family rented the video, *Hello, My Name is Bill.* It is the biography of Bill Wilson, the founder of Alcoholics Anonymous. I remember almost nothing about it except this scene. After Bill had overcome his own alcoholism, he kept leaving at all hours of the night to go help other men. At one point in her frustration, his wife asked something like, "Why do you keep giving so much of your time to a bunch of drunks, several of whom will never be thankful or stop drinking?" To this Bill replied, "Don't you know, I help them so I can stay sober." Giving to other sufferers will help each of them and you.

As a nurse, you now have a double gift to soothe people. I was glad to hear that you are already helping many, but look for additional opportunities to pass along comfort that you now know about first-hand. You have now been through that University of Hard Knocks and can speak from experience. Suggesting to other sufferers what might soothe physical discomforts or emotional upheavals will be like giving them a gift. Helping to feed the faith of other sufferers will make your own faith stronger. Reaching out can boost both of you.

I have a friend name Leland. Between surgery and chemo, Leland and his wife came to visit me. I told them that I was afraid of the imminent chemo. Leland said that since I had been such a good teacher, to look on this experience as intensive teacher training, getting me ready to help other people. When I was finished with chemo and back at worship, another lady in our congregation was diagnosed with breast cancer. She told Leland that I had already been a big help to her. Leland looked at me and said, "See, I knew you would!"

For several months I wrote to a lady named Kay who had advanced colon cancer and was a friend of my sister Twyla. Kay and I never met, but with Twyla's updates and by receiving one letter from Kay, I felt as if I knew her. I admired many things I heard about her. When I found out that she had problems with her gums or mouth, I told her about Magic Mouthwash. When I found out how much she was pushing herself to do, I encouraged her to pretend that she was her own child. Kay never recovered from her cancer, but she was still a victor in many ways. A week after Kay died, I received a letter from her husband's sister. This lady told me that the night Kay died, her husband searched to find her letters from me. He knew that they had been a spiritual comfort to Kay, and he wanted to read them too. I tell you this so that you will not underestimate the power of your own fitly spoken words at the proper time.

Proverbs 25:11 "A word aptly spoken is like apples of gold in settings of silver." (NIV) May God truly bless your health, your focus, your words, and those hands of yours that serve.

Your Sister in Christ,

Lynette

Alexander, one of the young men in our congregation recently led a prayer in which he asked God to help each of us "come up to the position of a servant." By using this incongruous combination of words, Alexander said volumes. The position of servant is down, not up, but Alexander knew that a servant for Christ lowers himself to be like the Savior. Without the Savor we might be exalted for a little while down here on earth, but what would we be in eternity? Yes, the "first will be last, and the last will be first." To want to serve others like Jesus did is to "come up" to the noble attitude of a humble love.

Dear Leah,

An expert in the law asked Jesus, "Who is my neighbor?" This prompted Jesus to tell the story of the Good Samaritan. The account includes conspicuously religious people who make the wrong choices as contrasted to a man who was an outcast to Jesus' audience. However, it is the social reject whom Jesus praises for his sympathetic actions. How memorable would this man have been if he had only good intentions? Instead, he gave his time, his first-aid supplies, his muscle, his transportation, his money, his compassion, and some of his future toward the care of this man from a race that hated the care giver.

Aesop told the story of a miser who buried his gold in a secret place. Every day he went to that spot, dug up the treasure and counted it. A thief observed him, then came back and dug up the treasure. When the miser discovered his loss, he was very upset. A neighbor heard his cries and asked what had happened. "Someone robbed me!" The neighbor asked why the man did not keep his gold in the house where he could easily get to it when he needed to buy things. "Buy things!" screamed the miser. "I would never spend any of that gold!" The neighbor then reached down and picked up a rock and threw it into the hole. "Then you might as well have just a rock in the hole. It is worth just as much to you as the treasure you lost," he said. The moral is that a possession is worth no more than the use one makes of it. A person who has the ability to help or comfort some sick person, but does not use that treasure, might as well have it taken away.

II Corinthians 1:3-4: "Praise be to the God and Father of our Lord Jesus Christ, the Father of compassion and the God of all comfort, who comforts us in all our troubles, so that we can comfort those in any trouble with the comfort we ourselves have received from God." (NIV)

In Him,

Lynette

This is a letter to my Maryville pharmacist.

Dear Don,

Thank you for going the "second mile" to get me medicine I needed. Most of all, I appreciate you being so accommodating that I do not have to add to my list of troubles, worrying over whether the medicine can be found. It also helps me to know that I do not have multiple pharmacists who are "here today and gone tomorrow," filling my prescriptions. I am often praying to God that He will give me comfort. One of the ways He sends His comfort is through kindnesses such as yours. I appreciate you, Roberta, and your employees.

Thank you,

Lynette

Dear Jan,

I was pleasantly surprised to receive the four caps you made me. They are especially good to sleep in, since they are so soft. Your caps can also be worn under a stiffer hat, since I have no hair to hang out around my face and neck. I also very much appreciate your specific prayers for me.

Love,

Lynette

My name was on the prayer list for ten months, often followed by the phrase, "She would appreciate cards." Yet in our congregation, there were people that I had known for fifteen years or thirty years, who never sent me a card or called. They missed an easy opportunity to symbolically give that cup of cold water to the Lord. However, it is the positive I choose to emphasize. I revel in the fact that several people reached out to me who hardly even knew me. These comforters initiated through calls, food, gifts, and letters.

One Sunday night, about four months before I found my cancer, as I was walking into the church building, I introduced myself to a lady I did not know. I had seen her previously from a distance on Sunday mornings. She told me her name was Ann, and she had recently moved to Knoxville. Four months later when I asked the congregation to pray for my upcoming surgery, it was Ann who called to say she would be driving twenty-five miles to bring us food. She had been through this twelve years earlier. Like me, she had been jerked off hormone replacements. By example, Ann taught me a very important thing: do not take a patient farther down the experience than she is that day, unless it is to give her genuine hope. She listened well, and she responded specifically to what I had just said. Ann spoke sympathetically and truly understood.

Several decades ago the renowned religious author J. B. Phillips wrote, "While I am certain that sickness is from the devil, I find it difficult to imagine how so many people would become motivated to reach out to others without sickness." As I was getting over my surgery, many members of the Ladies Bible Class volunteered to bring

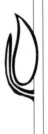

Even if you have not had extended illness yourself, you can be a comforter.

food. This was skillfully coordinated by two ladies named Mary and Frankie. Even if you have not had extended illness yourself, you can be a comforter. Do not limit yourself to vague volunteerism; that leaves the sick person having to ask for help. Jump right in and volunteer something. Quite a few years ago, an article appeared in *Readers' Digest* about a helpful man. Whenever there was a death in the family of one of his friends, he would show up with his shoe shine kit, saying, "Hi, I'm here to shine your shoes." He knew that people would want to look nice for the funeral. He also realized that in some circumstances there is little a person can say that will really help, so he decided to jump right in and show his concern. One grieving man tells that as he suffered with the death of a loved one, someone came and changed the oil in his car. When this easy chore seemed too taxing to accomplish, someone's simple kindness spoke volumes.

Regarding food: if a person is on chemo, do not make him any pungent dishes; avoid garlic, Parmesan cheese, or aromatic foods unless you know the person's nose and stomach can handle the fragrance. If the person is on chemo, do not prepare raw fruits or raw vegetables. Immunity will be low, and all bacteria cannot be completely washed off. Use canned fruits and vegetables or cook them. If you have sent raw fruit, do not kick yourself; the family of the sick person could eat it. It seems some people think that in order to take food to a sick person, one must take an entire meal. This is not always necessary. Some ladies pair up to make meals, or as you cook for your family, divide the casserole, baking it in two smaller dishes, giving half to the sick person's family. Do not give the family of the patient such a large quantity of a food that they will be tired of it before they can eat it all. Save containers that will be good for transporting foods. My friend Caroline saved glass jars to transport her homemade soup.

Regarding the gift of plants, at the time of surgery plants are a good idea, but if a person is in the midst of chemo, do not send flowers or a plant. They harbor bacteria that can be dangerous to a chemo patient. Morgan took all our plants to his office for four months. Again, do not be embarrassed if you have sent plants to a person in the midst of chemo. I am sure they looked at your love in action.

Regarding gifts, they come in all price ranges. My cousin Jan used her serger to make me four caps in ribbed cotton jersey. They were comfortable to sleep in and easy to wash and dry. I wore them daily for six months. Some people bought me books or loaned me books. Sharing the cost of a gift book with another person not only divides the expense, but also puts more people into the sick person's life. The type books that most appealed to me were books with short and uplifting sections. Do not give a book unless you have read it or know that it is recommended by Christians in those same circumstances. If you know the person's musical tastes, music is a very good gift. I especially enjoyed hymns and gospel songs. The best ones were full of hope, heaven, and words about God's love. Be aware that some "Christian" music goes against what the Bible teaches. Know the songs you are giving. The gift of taking the children of the patient to school or appointments is very appreciated. As I began to be able to get out again, my friend Beverly gave me the gift of being my chauffeur and the distraction of being taken on walks through flowering spring gardens. Get creative. Tape a worship service for your friend. Record yourself reading aloud something that you know your friend would enjoy. Send an audio letter, or make an audio scrapbook with one tape of messages from several friends. Arrange this in advance so each person can plan what she wants to say. Visit the patient wearing a weird hat and a costume. Other gift ideas include: humor books, a bed jacket, straws, videos, classic radio tapes, bed sheets, a special interest magazine, night clothes, postage stamps, or Cetaphil fragrance-free moisturizing cream. A lady named Johanna gave me a pill case that looked like a pocket watch. It is both cute and useful.

During the months between surgery and when chemo's effects ended, I could not handle complicated or challenging activities. However, I have a friend who while on chemo worked intricate puzzles. Know the patient's current capabilities or needs. Seeing my needs, my husband gave me a gift that has been used for countless hours. Because of bone pain at the end of my spine, my husband ordered a pillow that has a semi-circle cut out of the back so my spine never touches the seat of the

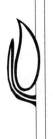

...do not forget to care for the care giver.

chair. He also ordered a fluffy cover for my seat belt so it would not press on me. Catalogs of comfort products: ALSTO'S (www.alsto.com or 1-800-447-0048); A.J. PRINDLE (www.ajprindle.com or 1-866-774-8278); INTELIHEALTH (www.ihcatalog.com or 1-800-988-1127); IMPROVE-MENTS at (www.ImprovementsCatalog.com or 1-800-642-2212) or the Preston Sammons Catalog. In addition, do not forget to care for the care giver.

Regarding cards, I recommend that you keep on hand a variety of get well cards with some being serious, others funny, and some Biblical. Often blank cards are best, so you can write your own sentiments. They should not all say, "Get Well." Some I received were more to lift the spirts.

At Thanksgiving, Christmas, Easter, and Mother's Day, cards came from people who wanted to let me know they were still praying for me, but chose to change from sending another get well card. Some people made me computer cards. My son Caleb sent me an art card he had crafted. Including handwritten personal messages is the best. When sending cards to a hospitalized person, put his own home address on the envelope's upper left corner. If the patient is dismissed from the hospital, his own return address will still get the card to him. I keep a variety of new cards and file them by topic. I also recommend that you make a notebook or a computer file of scriptures, quotes, poems, stories, and encouragements to uplift people. Each could be categorized for different struggles such as extended illness, injury, depression, bereavement, or the joy of recovery. If the person has an extended illness or chronic health problems, mark your calendar to send him a card each Tuesday, each Friday, or find out his chemo calendar and schedule your cards to him to arrive on a certain day after treatments. Predictability will give the patient something to anticipate.

Dear John,

One day in January, two cards arrived that were both from G.C. and Mattie Lou. One card was theologically deep and wise. The other card was drawn cartoon-style with a rumpled man standing in the rain holding a broken umbrella and the leash of an uncooperative dog. It said, "There are some people who say we can learn a lot from times like these—wouldn't you like to smack 'em?!" I inferred from the cards that G.C. and Mattie Lou were saying they knew how distressing and difficult the ordeal was, but they hoped I was finding a few things to give me a chuckle. May you also find chuckles.

Yours truly,

Lynette

I have enclosed parts of letters I received from a lady named Belinda. Besides the Lord, she and I had little in common. We knew one another only slightly until 1999 when we served on a church committee together. Several things we had to discuss at length caused me to see Belinda from new perspectives. I think she probably gained new appreciations of me also. Even though we still have little in common, it no longer matters, because we have seen and heard one another's hearts speak. She wrote me articulate, poignant, picturesque letters sprinkled with Bible verses.

Dear Lynette,

You are on my mind so I wanted to spend some time in prayer for you and in the Word with you in mind. I continue to pray for your complete healing and that your body be cancer-free. I believe God hears the prayers of His faithful and adds years to their lives. In response to my reading of Isaiah 38, my prayer is: "Remember, O Lord, how Lynette has walked before You faithful and with whole-hearted devotion and has done what is good in Your eyes."

I pray also for your spirit, that you may experience peace, joy, hope, and love in your inner being and be strengthened and comforted by His promises and faithfulness.

Isaiah 43:2: "When you pass through the waters, I will be with you; and through the rivers, they will not overflow you. When you walk through the fire, you shall not be burned; nor shall the flame scorch you."

Psalm 23: "Though I walk through the valley of the shadow of death, I will fear no evil, for You are with me." And Psalm 56: "You have put all my tears in Your bottle; are they not in Your book? In God I have put my trust; I will not be afraid."

Deep water, valleys, tears and fears are inevitable, but praise God that He is the WHO there with us in the WHEN.

I pray that you maintain an outlook that chemo is your ally in this fight, and that "this too shall pass." Remember that hair will grow back, but every cancer cell that dies is dead forever. Psalm 69 prompts this prayer for you: "Do not let the flood waters engulf Lynette or the pit close its mouth over her. Answer her, O Lord, out of the goodness of your love."

I love you, as does your whole church family. We are on the sidelines cheering you on in your race, saying "Run Lynette, Run!"

My Love in Him,

Belinda

Dear Cayce,

Now that chemo is behind you, I can mention things that were not timely to bring up earlier. Some days I look back on all that I went through in connection to cancer, and I cannot believe that I really did endure. Then I can hardly believe that I have flourished in spite of all my struggles, fears, the normal digestive problems, anemia, my immunity and stamina being bombarded, and being crippled by adverse reaction to drugs. I am proud that I have overcome. Since you also have come through more than you ever thought possible, pat yourself on the back. You deserve it. Nevertheless, in spite of what I have overcome, I know that it was God enabling and empowering this wimp. If tomorrow any trouble comes knocking on my door again, I would have to learn these lessons all over again. The difference would be that this time I would have experience, having already relied on God and succeeded, therefore I should remember to look for His strength again.

Both of my sons have been storytellers. They have entertained hundreds with the adventures they tell from children's literature. Most of their pieces include a variety of voices, accents, and characters, along with a contrast of gestures and expressions. Some of the stories which my older son told eight years ago he no longer remembers, but he can read certain children's books three or four times and have the story fall right into place again. His mind and body remember having said those sequences of words and put together those arrangements of movements; they remember having become a frog, a space alien, or a wolf.

Of course, I pray for your good health, but even more than that, I pray for you the same things that I pray for me—that we will be spiritually minded, adaptable, able to laugh, observant, and wanting to work with God.

Love,

Lynette

This is to my childhood friend whom I have not seen in forty years. I still think of her as the girl who loved to laugh, sing, play the piano, and visit the Dairy Dip.

Dear Barbara,

So much has happened since exactly two years ago when we each discovered cancer. I came out of chemo looking whiter than paste, worn, and fatigued. Because I am so atypical, adjuvant care brought me rigorous ailments and muscle atrophy. However, a few weeks ago, as I was out in the garden of our neighbors Herb and Sybil, I contemplated what it meant that I was shucking corn, picking crowder peas, and running each pod through the sheller. Other days I am in weight training or being a Bible class teacher. I realized how very far I have come since cancer. My body, mind, heart, and spirit have learned so much. Unlike some people, I don't think I will ever be able to briefly mention "cancer's benefits"; it is such an oxymoron that those two words need much more explanation when used in tandem. Even so, I know that cancer can be one of life's teachers. What a person learns depends on her experiences and willingness to search for meanings. Cancer has taught me to exercise more, eat better, investigate health in depth, research even the recommendations of doctors, but to have my focus be spiritual. It also taught me to prioritize with Godly perspective, not worldly emphasis. I have found many blessings that came along with cancer, through cancer, because of cancer, or in spite of cancer, but they did not come because the struggle was easy or the lessons were spelled out. God showered down enrichments then and now because I leaned, searched, asked, sought, knocked, prayed, read, researched, and vowed that this experience would not be in vain.

You were the first person to whom I wrote, and you were the first person who encouraged me to write a book. Therefore, it is only fitting that my book should end by writing to you. An unknown author wrote that story which I told you twenty months ago about the little girl who wanted to help another. I have included sending it to the majority of the forty people to whom I have sent letters.

A little girl arrived home later than usual. Her mother asked her why she was so late. The little girl told her mother, "I had to stop to help another girl, because she was in trouble."

"What did you do to help her?" the mother asked.

"Oh, I sat down and helped her cry."

Yes, I hope I have sympathetically helped you and many other sufferers cry tears of commiseration, tears of joy, and tears of hope. The journey through crisis can truly lead to great enhancements.

Love,

Lynette

for further
thought

for further thought

1. What is the theme of Luke 22:27; Matthew 20:28; and Ephesians 5:21?

2. Explain the value of Dr. Karl Menninger's advice to help others.

3. Tell specifically what benevolence cost the Good Samaritan in Luke 10:25-37.

4. What is the use of an ability that we never use?

5. At judgment when God is dividing the sheep from the goats, when He tells His sheep that they have given Him a drink or visited, who is it that they had fed or visited? (Matthew 25:31-46)

6. How is Ann's advice to not take a patient down the road further than she is that day similar to Matthew 6:34?

7. Analyze the statement by J.B. Phillips, "While I am certain that sickness is from the devil, I find it difficult to imagine how so many people would become motivated to reach out to others without sickness."

8. Why is specific volunteerism better than vaguely offering to help? Could your specifics be too inflexible?

9. Write out a few verses, quotes, or sentiments that you would use to send someone with prolonged illness.

10. How can a book or tape be the worst gift or the best gift for a struggler?

11. Why is it wise to make a file of scriptures, quotes, and poems to uplift the injured, sick, or grieving?

12. How is giving joy like a boomerang?

Appendix
Suggestions for Supplies

Recommended Books
Recommended Music
Healthier Recipes

SUGGESTIONS OF SUPPLIES DURING SURGERY, CHEMO, OR RADIATION

SPIRAL NOTEBOOK: Include phone numbers of doctors, pharmacy, relatives, and helpful friends; questions to ask the doctor; doctor's answers; jargon; list gifts and food brought; when thank yous were sent; list drugs taken and their schedule; write down precious remarks said; compose an original prayer.

LETTER HOLDER OR BOX: A place exclusively for get well cards sent to you

GALLON SIZE ZIP-LOCK BAGS: These are good for cards you received in previous weeks.

BASKET: Choose a size to hold all your regular bath time toiletries plus those for your new physical needs.

SATCHEL OR STURDY BAG: This is to take to chemo and hold all that you need there.

MUSIC PLAYER: This could be a CD player and CD or a cassette player and tape. I took one for me and one for Morgan. The television in the chemo room was often on something we did not want to watch.

SOFT CAPS: If you lose your hair, these caps are good for around the house and to sleep in. Choose styles with nothing to hurt your head as you lie on them and styles that are easy to launder.

THANK YOU CARDS OR BLANK NOTES: Have more than one type.

POSTAGE STAMPS

THERMOMETER: Elevated temperature can indicate infection.

FLASHLIGHT: Small size to keep by the bed when getting up at night.

HEATING PAD AND/OR HOT WATER BOTTLE: When the weather is cool this can be a comfort. When trying to find a vein this will also help.

HUMIDIFIER: Chemo administered during winter months may dry the nose. Choose an easy to clean model.

"COLD CARE" KLEENEX or LOTION PUFFS TISSUE: Fragrance-free and softer than most.

CETAPHIL: Fragrance-free moisturizing cream even for people with allergies.

KERI or CUREL: Fragrance-free lotion.

HUGGIES BABY WIPES: Choose the variety that is fragrance-free (for digestive tract sensitivities).

BALMEX or DESITIN: Chemo can affect the digestive tract anywhere from beginning to end.

AYR: Saline nasal mist or gel for dry nose.

VITAMIN E OIL: Helps a surgery wound.

ANTI-BACTERIAL SWABS: To administer Vitamin E oil to a surgery wound or to administer Vitamin E to dry nostrils. Be careful to never contaminate the swab or the oil.

BENDABLE STRAWS: Chemo drugs may dry out lips.

LIP LUBRICANT: Chapstick may be very relieving, but be very aware that certain fragrances may bother you on specific days. Health food stores sell types without petroleum.

TOOTHBRUSHES: Buy several with a smaller head and very soft bristles. Change your toothbrush every three weeks to thwart germs. Some patients like a battery powered model with a tiny round head. Keep it off hurting gums.

"GENTLE CARE" WOVEN FLOSS: A loosely braided cotton to protect gums.

MAGIC MOUTHWASH: This is one of several prescriptions for raw gums and throat. Swish, gargle, or swallow this thick pain-killer that thwarts infection.

FIRST AID GAUZE AND TAPE: This is for people putting oil or medicine on a surgery wound. This will keep clothes from getting stained.

SENNA-S: This is an over-the-counter stool softener that may be needed immediately following surgery.

IMODIUM D: Chemo may cause diarrhea on certain days. The liquid type works faster, but if you are at least two months into chemo, the liquid may sting your esophagus, therefore, later in your treatments the tablet form may be easier to swallow.

DEODORANT: During radiation, use cornstarch in a shaker or use Arm and Hammer with Baking Soda; Tom's of Maine; or Alba Botanica.

"What we suffer now is nothing compared to the glory He will give us later."

—Romans 8:18

RECOMMENDED BOOKS FOR THE PHYSICAL

AMERICAN CANCER SOCIETY'S GUIDE TO COMPLEMENTARY AND ALTERNATIVE CANCER METHODS ISBN: 0-944235-24-7 This encyclopedic book is divided into sections, some of which are very useful and others that are not. The beginning discusses connections between the mind, physical touch, and healing and explains aromatherapy to Transcutaneous Electrical Nerve Stimulation. Other sections are on herbs, vitamins, minerals, diet, nutrition, and biological treatments. Each article tells how that substance is promoted, what is its history, the scientific evidence, and possible complications.

THE BREAST CANCER PREVENTION DIET by Bob Arnot MD. ISBN: 0-316-05109-8 This comprehensive and easy to read book is structured so that a person can read only the chapters of her choice.

HOW TO REDUCE YOUR RISK OF BREAST CANCER by Jon J. Michnovicz MD, Ph.D. ISBN: 0-446-67104-5 This book explains the risk factors. It has sections on estrogen, dietary fat, eating fruits and vegetables, and phytochemicals.

A PERFECT 10: PHYTO "NEW-TRIENTS" AGAINST CANCERS by Dr. Laura Pawlak PhD, RD. This easy to understand book focuses on specific foods to eat if your want to prevent getting certain cancers.

RECOMMENDED BOOKS FOR THE SPIRITUAL

DISRUPTED: Finding God in Illness and Loss by Virgil Fry. ISBN 0-89098-252-X The chaplain at M.D. Anderson Cancer Center shares experiences, quotes, and prayers.

EVERYDAY STRENGTH: A Cancer Patient's Guide by Randy Becton. ISBN: 0-8010-0975-8 A Christian man who has suffered through cancer writes with sympathy and practicality using scripture, suggestions, and prayer.

THOSE WHO WAIT by Rosemary McKnight. ISBN: 0-89225-365-7 Isaiah 40:31 is the text for this simple book that is soothing for those who wait on God, wait for answers, and wait for time to pass during any type struggle. McKnight discusses how waiting can be hopeful, active, and instructive.

RECOMMENDED MUSIC

IMAGES OF GOD, VOLUME V by Jeff Nelson. (Howard Publishing 1-800-858-4109) 20 songs from the hymnal, *Songs of Faith and Praise* include: "My Eyes Are Dry," "Listen to Our Hearts," "Like a River," "How Beautiful," "Breath of Heaven," "I Am a Sheep," "Come Share the Lord," "Who Can Satisfy My Soul Like You?"

WALKING IN SUNLIGHT by Ray Walker. (Dallas Christian Sound 1-800-654-5918) Both usual and unusual arrangements of 22 well-loved hymns such as: "On Jordan's Stormy Banks," "No Tears in Heaven," "In the Sweet By and By," "Be With Me Lord," "O Lord, Our Lord," "The Ninety and Nine," "Near to the Heart of God," "Standing On the Promises," "As the Life of a Flower," and "When They Ring Those Golden Bells."

WE SHALL RISE by Dedication. (1-615 228-2926) 10 songs include: "We Shall Rise," "Sweet Sweet Spirit," "God is My Rock," "River of Jordan," "The Lord's My Shepherd," and "If That Isn't Love."

WORSHIP HIS GLORY IN ACAPPELLA PRAISE by The Cathedrals. (1-800-827-2936) 14 songs including: "Just a Little Talk With Jesus," "There is a Fountain," "He Keeps Me Singing." "Down By the Riverside," "I Am Bound For the Promised Land," "Shall We Gather at the River," "When We All Get to Heaven. "

CDs from Christian universities' choral groups

"He has put a new song in my mouth, a hymn of praise to our God."

—Psalm 40:3

HEALTHIER RECIPES

These are recipes I have originated or altered to contain less fat; higher fiber; no growth hormones, antibiotics, or dyes; and to emphasize fruits and vegetables. Other ideas that you can try are:

Use more **brown rice** instead of white, and use **whole grain pastas**.

Add additional vegetables to any can of **soup** you open or to homemade soup.

Into the **sauce** for spaghetti or lasagna, stir in shredded carrots and/or fresh parsley.

Emphasize dark greens such as spinach for **tossed salads**.

Top a **tossed salad** with mandarin oranges, dried cherries, or dried cranberries.

Top a **tossed salad** with some drained whole kernel corn or pecans or walnuts.

When making your favorite **cornbread**, stir in a box of chopped broccoli.

Buy a large container of organic **yogurt** and each day top one serving with a different fruit.

When making large amounts of **meatloaf or sloppy joes**, stir in mashed black-eyed peas.

Instead of butter or margarine on **baked potatoes**, try them with chili that you have made with less meat (preferably organic) and more beans (both kidney beans and black beans).

When making **mashed potatoes,** omit or limit butter or margarine, and instead use plain organic yogurt, dry organic milk, and water. Or, use organic low-fat sour cream.

When making a **brownie mix** that calls for 2 eggs, ½ cup of oil, and 1/4 cup water, INSTEAD substitute these: 1 egg, 1/4 cup canola oil, 1/3 cup organic yogurt, 4 ounce jar of baby food plums, prunes OR sweet potatoes, 2 tablespoons of wheat bran, and 1/4 cup water.

Ask your produce manager if he can get **broccolini**. It is more tender, less bitter, and has less waste than broccoli. Dip 3 seconds into boiling water. Drain. Chill. Eat.

BLUEBERRY SALAD

2 envelopes of unflavored/unsweetened gelatin

Stir gelatin into 1/2 cup of COOL water; stir; dissolve.

1 cup boiled water

While this water is in a rolling boil, add the gelatin/cool water gel. Stir. Remove from heat. Add 4 ice cubes. Stir.

1 can blueberry pie filling (Choose a brand with no added dye.)

20 oz. can crushed pineapple, undrained

Mix all ingredients. Refrigerate. Congeal.

(Sometimes I even add extra blueberries to make it fruit dense. Option: use peach, cherry, or blackberry pie filling.)

BROCCOLI SALAD

(No raw produce while on chemo. Adjust the amounts according to your tastes and needs.)

1 head of fresh broccoli, chopped

3-6 cups of water

Boil water. Immerse broccoli for 3 SECONDS. This will brighten it. Drain WELL.

1/3 cup dry roasted sunflower kernels OR 1/3 cup **dry roasted** peanuts

1/2 cup raisins OR 1 cup grapes

Mix broccoli, sunflower kernels, & fruit. In a separate bowl, mix the dressing.

Dressing:

1/3 cup organic yogurt

2 tablespoons sugar

1 tablespoon apple cider vinegar

Pour the dressing over the broccoli mixture. Toss and chill. Does not store well overnight.

HEALTHY SLAW

(Not for anyone currently on chemo; no raw produce then.)

Shredded cabbage

Shredded carrots

Organic yogurt

1-2 tablespoon sugar

1-2 tablespoons orange juice concentrate

1 tablespoon lemon juice (optional)

Mix. For color and texture, add diced apples, grapes, OR mandarin oranges.

CRANBERRY AND APPLE CASSEROLE

1-2 apples, sliced

1 can whole berry cranberry sauce

3/4 cup oats

1/3 cup nuts, chopped (walnuts or pecans)

1/2 cup fresh or frozen cranberries (optional)

1/3 cup brown sugar

1/4 cup flour

1/3 cup juice (choose cranberry OR grape OR apple OR orange; each gives different flavor)

Put apple slices on bottom of glass casserole dish. Top with cranberry sauce. If you have them, toss on the fresh or frozen cranberries. In a different bowl, mix all the dry ingredients. Sprinkle oat mixture over the fruit. Last, drizzle with juice of your choice. Bake at 325 degrees for 20-25 minutes. Good for breakfast, lunch, dinner, or even topped with frozen yogurt for dessert. I often double this recipe.

HEALTHY SHAKE

8 oz. organic plain yogurt (1 cup) Have all ingredients very cold.

1/2 cup calcium fortified orange juice

2 tablespoon dry powdered organic milk

1 large carrot sliced OR 4 baby carrots sliced

3/4 cup frozen or fresh fruit (strawberries, banana, blueberries, raspberries, or peaches)

1 tablespoon flax seeds that have been freshly ground up

2 tablespoons wheat germ and/or wheat bran

Put ingredients in blender. Blend on low and then increase the speed to high for 1-2 minutes depending on the type machine you have. Makes enough for 2 drinks.

(Sometimes I omit the orange juice and use 1/4 cup grape juice **concentrate** and 1/4 cup milk.

Some people will want to add 1 to 2 tablespoons of sugar or honey.)

CINNAMON APPLES

6-8 apples

2 tablespoons lemon juice

3 tablespoons water

Arrange sliced apples in Pyrex dish. Pour lemon juice/water mixture over apples.

3/4 cup sugar

1 1/2 teaspoons cinnamon

1/2 cup flour

salt (optional)

1 cup organic cheese (American or cheddar) shredded

In a dry bowl mix remaining ingredients. Pour dry mixture over apples. Drizzle with 1/4 cup fruit juice (apple, cranberry, or orange) Bake 25-30 minutes at 325-350 degrees. Let rest a few minutes before eating.

PEDRO'S SPECIAL

1 onion chopped

1 pound Laura's Lean ground beef (Organic: no growth hormones or antibiotic)

1 clove garlic (optional)

Brown in large skillet. Drain on paper towel (with no color on the paper). Swab out skillet. Put meat mixture back in skillet. Add:

16 oz. can diced tomatoes

8 oz. can tomato sauce

16 oz. can kidney beans

16 oz can black beans (OR can of whole kernel corn, drained)

1/4 teaspoon chopped oregano

1 or 2 Tablespoons chili powder

Stir. Heat. Stir. Serve as is. OR serve on top of baked potatoes. OR put in a large glass baking dish and top with:

1/2 cup organic cheese, shredded

1/2 cup BAKED corn chips, smashed (optional)

Bake 350 degrees for 25 minutes.

MEAT BALLS

2 pounds of Laura's Lean ground beef

1/3 cup dry organic milk

2/3 cup oats

1/2 can black-eyed peas, mashed

1 egg

1/3 cup onion, finely chopped

1/4 teaspoon garlic powder

dash salt

pepper (optional)

1 teaspoon chili powder

Combine all ingredients. Shape into balls the size of a walnut. Place close together in a Pyrex dish you have sprayed with oil. Pour sauce over top. Bake at 325 degrees for 30-40 minutes.

Sauce: 2 cups of catsup

1/2 cup brown sugar

1/4 teaspoon garlic powder

1/4 cup chopped onion

ELECTRIC SKILLET SLOPPY JOES

3/4 cup fresh onion, chopped

1 pound Laura's Lean ground beef (Organic: No hormones, no antibiotics like other beef)

Brown beef in onions. Drain on paper towel (with no printing). Swab out skillet.

16 oz. can black-eyed peas (Luck's Fat-free black-eyed peas have no preservatives.)

Mash peas well and they are undetectable. Place beef and mashed peas in skillet. Add:

1 1/2 cups catsup & 2 cups of water

2 tablespoons apple cider vinegar

2 tablespoons lemon juice

2 tablespoons brown sugar

1 tablespoon prepared mustard

Stir gently to not have it go over the edge.

Simmer on medium heat in electric skillet **with the lid on it** for 30 minutes. Then as you cook it for about 20 more minutes, continually check on it every 5 minutes to make sure it has not cooked out all the liquid. I usually have to gradually add **more** water. I cook it until all the additional water has been absorbed.

CARROT CAKE

2 cups of sugar

1 cup of canola oil

2/3 cup applesauce OR organic yogurt

3 eggs (Eggland's brand contains Omega-3 fatty acid, beneficial to health.)

2 cups unbleached all-purpose flour

1/4 cup oats

2 teaspoons baking soda

1 teaspoon salt

2 teaspoons cinnamon

3 1/2 cups coarsely grated raw carrots (Shredded in food processor)

1 cup walnuts OR pecans

Preheat oven to 300 degrees. Combine first 4 ingredients. Beat at medium speed for 2 minutes. Add dry ingredients and beat on low speed for 1 minute. Stir in carrots and nuts. Spread batter in 9x13 inch pan that has been oiled. Bake at 300 degrees for 1 hour, until cake tests done with toothpick.

FOUR TOPPING OPTIONS from which to choose:

(1) Top with warmed pineapple and its juice.

(2) Make sauce with: ½ cup sugar, 1 Tablespoon cornstarch; 1 cup boiling water; vanilla.

(3) Dust with powdered sugar.

(4) Make a frosting of organic cream cheese, vanilla, organic milk, and confectioners sugar. Soften cream cheese in microwave by heating on lower setting for a few seconds. Add milk only as needed; a little goes a long way. Smash ingredients together with fork and stir.